Communications
in Computer and Information Science   982

Commenced Publication in 2007
Founding and Former Series Editors:
Phoebe Chen, Alfredo Cuzzocrea, Xiaoyong Du, Orhun Kara, Ting Liu,
Krishna M. Sivalingam, Dominik Ślęzak, and Xiaokang Yang

More information about this series at http://www.springer.com/series/7899

Panagiotis D. Bamidis ·
Martina Ziefle · Leszek A. Maciaszek (Eds.)

Information and Communication Technologies for Ageing Well and e-Health

4th International Conference, ICT4AWE 2018
Funchal, Madeira, Portugal, March 22–23, 2018
Revised Selected Papers

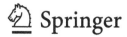 Springer

Editors
Panagiotis D. Bamidis
Aristotle University of Thessaloniki
Thessaloniki, Greece

Leeds Institute of Medical Education
University of Leeds
Leeds, UK

Leszek A. Maciaszek
Wrocław University of Economics
Institute of Business Informatics
Wrocław, Poland

Macquarie University
Department of Computing
Sydney, NSW, Australia

Martina Ziefle
Institut für Psychologie
RWTH Aachen University
Aachen, Nordrhein-Westfalen, Germany

ISSN 1865-0929   ISSN 1865-0937 (electronic)
Communications in Computer and Information Science
ISBN 978-3-030-15735-7   ISBN 978-3-030-15736-4 (eBook)
https://doi.org/10.1007/978-3-030-15736-4

Library of Congress Control Number: 2019934738

This Springer imprint is published by the registered company Springer Nature Switzerland AG
The registered company address is: Gewerbestrasse 11, 6330 Cham, Switzerland

Preface

The present book includes extended and revised versions of a set of selected papers from the 4th International Conference on Information and Communication Technologies for Ageing Well and e-Health (ICT4AWE 2018), held in Funchal, Madeira, Portugal, during March 22–23, 2018.

We received 51 paper submissions from 20 countries, of which 20% are included in this book. The papers were selected by the event chairs and their selection is based on a number of criteria that include the classifications and comments provided by the Program Committee members, the session chairs' assessment and also the program chairs' global view of all papers included in the technical program. The authors of selected papers were then invited to submit a revised and extended version of their papers having at least 30% innovative material.

The International Conference on Information and Communication Technologies for Ageing Well and e-Health aims to be an international meeting point for those that study and apply information and communication technologies for improving the quality of life of the elderly and for helping people stay healthy, independent, and active at work or in their community along their whole life. ICT4AWE facilitates the exchange of information and dissemination of best practices, innovation, and technical improvements in the fields of age-related health care, education, social coordination, and ambient assisted living. From e-health to intelligent systems, and ICT devices, this will be a point of interest for all those working in research and development and in companies involved in promoting the well-being of aged people, by providing room for industrial presentations, demos and project descriptions.

The ten papers selected to be included in this book contribute to the understanding of relevant trends of current research on information and communication technologies for ageing well and e-health: The topics covered by the authors show clearly the major cornerstones in the development and design of timely and human-centered approaches in a variety of usage contexts. In their contribution, Eva-Maria Schomakers and colleagues show how older adults can be integrated by personal and playful assessment of their acceptance of AAL technologies. In line with this, Wiktoria Wilkowska and her coauthors report on an empirical study in which older adults' trust and trustfulness in technical devices are explored as an important prerequisite for the devices' successful integration in home environments. The third study, authored by Julia Offermann-van Heek and colleagues, changes the perspective to caregivers and shows how care professionals perceive potential benefits and barriers of AAL technology usage. In a position paper, a group of eight researchers (Diotima Bertel et al.) expand on the concepts of engagement platforms and engagement ecosystems, arguing that an integration of physical and virtual worlds is necessary for AAL advisory services. In order to empower people's motivation to engage in physical activity at older age, another study (authored by Despoina Petsani and coworkers) introduces an multidisciplinary e-coaching approach (webFitForAll) that integrates new ideas from co-creation and co-design with the actual users. However, not only the devices themselves are in the focus, but also the question of how health-related information on websites can gain credibility and trust for older adults, as shown by Luisa Verviers and colleagues. In addition, ICT in health-related systems and devices are also useful for specific age-related diseases and shortcomings. Robin Amsters and his colleagues demonstrate a novel vision-based spatio-temporal gait analysis system using a mobile platform. As diabetes prevalence has steadily been increasing over the past decades in the older adults group, Andre Calero Valdez and coworkers developed and tested the user acceptance of Diabetto, a novel digital diabetes diary with interactive therapy support and access to a nutrition database through pen-input and text-to-speech. Another paper moves from the home context to urban and suburban transport ecosystems and examines the spread of service areas, accessibility of provided services, and availability of demand-driven services for older adults and persons with disabilities (authored by Stefan Ruscher and coworkers). The last paper in this book of selected papers is authored by Andreia Nunes and colleagues and is directed at the acceptance of mobile health applications, looking specifically at the role people's demographic and personality factors play in the behavioral intention to use mHealth apps.

We would like to thank all the authors for their contributions and also the reviewers who have helped ensure the quality of this publication.

March 2018   Panagiotis D. Bamidis
                                                                      Martina Ziefle
                                                              Leszek A. Maciaszek

Organization

Conference Chair

Leszek Maciaszek — Wroclaw University of Economics, Poland and Macquarie University, Sydney, Australia

Program Co-chairs

Panagiotis Bamidis — Aristotle University of Thessaloniki, Greece and Leeds Institute of Medical Education, University of Leeds, UK

Martina Ziefle — RWTH Aachen University, Germany

Program Committee

Mehdi Adda	Université du Québec à Rimouski, Canada
Kenji Araki	Hokkaido University, Japan
Carmelo Ardito	Università degli Studi di Bari, Italy
Christopher Baber	University of Birmingham, UK
Giacinto Barresi	Istituto Italiano di Tecnologia, Italy
Rashid Bashshur	Michigan Medicine, USA
Juan-Manuel Belda-Lois	Instituto de Biomecánica de València, Spain
Karsten Berns	Robotics Research Lab, Germany
Laurent Billonnet	Ensil-Ensci - Université de Limoges, France
Philipp Brauner	RWTH Aachen University, Germany
Jane Bringolf	Centre for Universal Design Australia Ltd., Australia
Yao Chang	Chung Yuan Christian University, Taiwan
Mario Ciampi	National Research Council of Italy, Italy
Malcolm Clarke	Brunel University, UK
Ana Correia de Barros	Fraunhofer Portugal AICOS, Portugal
Georg Duftschmid	Medical University of Vienna, Austria
Stefano Federici	University of Perugia, Italy
Ana Fred	Instituto de Telecomunicações and Instituto Superior Técnico, Lisbon University, Portugal
David Fuschi	BRIDGING Consulting Ltd., UK
Alastar Gale	Loughborough University, UK
Ennio Gambi	Università Politecnica delle Marche, Italy
Javier Gomez	Universidad Autonoma de Madrid, Spain
Florian Grond	McGill University, Canada
Jaakko Hakulinen	University of Tampere, Finland
Alina Huldtgren	Eindhoven University of Technology, The Netherlands

Eila Jarvenpaa	Aalto University, Finland
Petr Ježek	University of West Bohemia, Czech Republic
Takahiro Kawamura	Japan Science and Technology Agency, Japan
Peter Kokol	University of Maribor, Slovenia
Evdokimos Konstantinidis	Aristotle University of Thessaloniki, Greece
Mikel Larrea	Universidad del País Vasco, Spain
Christine Lisetti	Florida International University, USA
Ahmad Lotfi	Nottingham Trent University, UK
Jin Luo	London South Bank University, UK
Leszek Maciaszek	Wroclaw University of Economics, Poland and Macquarie University, Sydney, Australia
Heimar Marin	Universidade Federal de São Paulo, Brazil
Maurice Mars	University of KwaZulu-Natal, South Africa
Cezary Mazurek	Poznan Supercomputing and Networking Center, Poland
Elvis Mazzoni	University of Bologna, Italy
René Meier	Lucerne University of Applied Sciences, Switzerland
Iosif Mporas	University of Hertfordshire, UK
Maurice Mulvenna	Ulster University, UK
Anthony Norcio	University of Maryland Baltimore County, USA
Marko Perisa	University of Zagreb, Croatia
Zainab Pirani	MHSaboo Siddik College of Engineering, India
Marco Porta	Università degli Studi di Pavia, Italy
Amon Rapp	University of Turin, Italy
Ulrich Reimer	University of Applied Sciences St. Gallen, Switzerland
Philippe Roose	LIUPPA/IUT de Bayonne/UPPA, France
Corina Sas	Lancaster University, UK
Sreela Sasi	Gannon University, USA
Andreas Schrader	Universität zu Lübeck, Germany
Jitae Shin	Sungkyunkwan University, Korea, Republic of
Oh-Soon Shin	Soongsil University, Korea, Republic of
Josep Silva	Universitat Politècnica de València, Spain
Åsa Smedberg	Stockholm University, Sweden
Luca Spalazzi	Università Politecnica delle Marche, Italy
Susanna Spinsante	Università Politecnica delle Marche, Italy
Taro Sugihara	Okayama University, Japan
Babak Taati	Toronto Rehabilitation Institute, Canada
Andrew Targowski	Western Michigan University, USA
Carolyn Turvey	University of Iowa, USA
Bert-Jan van Beijnum	University of Twente, Netherlands
Andrea Vitaletti	Università degli Studi di Roma La Sapienza, Italy
Doug Vogel	Harbin Institute of Technology, China
Meng Wong	Education National Institute of Singapore, Singapore

George Xylomenos   Athens University of Economics and Business, Greece
Martina Ziefle   RWTH Aachen University, Germany
Evi Zouganeli   Oslo Metropolitan University, Norway

Additional Reviewer

Nikhil Deshpande   Istituto Italiano di Tecnologia, Italy

Invited Speakers

Patty Kostkova   University College London, UK
Giuseppe Conti   Nively, Italy

Contents

Influence of User Factors on the Acceptance of Ambient Assisted Living Technologies in Professional Care Contexts

Julia Offermann-van Heek[✉], Martina Ziefle, and Simon Himmel

Human-Computer Interaction Center, RWTH Aachen University,
52074 Aachen, Germany
vanheek@comm.rwth-aachen.de

Abstract. Demographic change in conjunction with increasing amounts of older people and people in need of care pose high burdens and challenges for the care sectors of today's society. In the last decades, it is tried to face these challenges by developing technical solutions in the area of Ambient Assisted Living (AAL). Besides technical functions and opportunities, the acceptance of future users is decisive for a successful implementation of those technologies in everyday life situations. As AAL technologies have an enormous potential to support care staff as well as caretakers in professional care situations, it is questionable to what extent professional care staff accepts and adopts to use assisting technologies in their professional everyday life. In more detail, it is of major interest to analyze how care professionals perceive potential benefits and barriers of AAL technology usage, specific characteristics of data gathering and storage as well as if individual user factors of care professionals influence the perception and acceptance of AAL technologies.

Keywords: Ambient assisted living technologies · Technology acceptance · Professional caregivers · User factors

1 Introduction

Increasing amounts of older people and people in need of care characterize demographic change and represent major challenges for today's society and the respective care sectors [1–3].

The consequences of demographic change become visible in diverse care areas: in particular, lack of care specialists in combination with higher proportions of old and ill people who have to be cared challenge geriatric and nursing care institutions [4–7]. Simultaneously, there is a comparably new phenomenon of a first generation of "old people with disabilities" – on the one hand, due to medical and technical developments in healthcare and, on the other hand, due to the specific historical background of euthanasia offenses (in particular in Europe), in which disabled people have been systematically deported or even murdered [8]. Thus, in accordance with the challenges for geriatric and nursing care, the sector of care and support of people with disabilities is also confronted with higher proportions of people in need of care with a

© Springer Nature Switzerland AG 2019
P. D. Bamidis et al. (Eds.): ICT4AWE 2018, CCIS 982, pp. 1–25, 2019.
https://doi.org/10.1007/978-3-030-15736-4_1

simultaneously existing lack of care specialists [9]. To sum up, these three care areas face essentially the same challenges and solutions have to be found to address those challenges.

For this purpose, technical innovations and ideas have been increasingly developed in the last years in order to relieve care staff, to enable a longer staying at the own home for older people, or to enhance safety in emergencies. These technical developments include technical single-case solutions as well as more complex ambient assisted living (AAL) systems [10, 11], aiming for a detecting of falls and emergencies, monitoring of vital parameters, or enabling a longer stay at the own home using smart home technology elements [12–15].

Besides a broad range of technical functions and opportunities, current research revealed that those systems are rarely used in real life – specifically in professional environments [16]. As the users' acceptance is necessary and decisive for a successful and sustainable implementation and usage of innovative assisting technologies, diverse stakeholders and their perceptions have to be addressed. For a successful implementation in professional care contexts, the opinions, ideas, and wishes of professional caregivers are decisive and should be investigated. Thus the current study focuses in particular on care professionals' perspectives on specific AAL technologies, on data gathering, data storage and access as well as perceived benefits and barriers of AAL technology usage. The results enable an integration of professional caregivers' perspectives into the design of AAL technologies and a better understanding of professional caregivers' requirements. This way, an adaption of those technologies to the needs and wishes of professional caregivers can be enabled and the usage of AAL technologies in professional care contexts can potentially be increased.

2 AAL Technologies in Professional Care Contexts

In the following section, the theoretical background of the current study is presented starting with a short overview of current AAL technologies and systems. Afterwards, the theoretical background of technology acceptance as well as results of previous acceptance studies in the context of AAL technologies used in professional care contexts are described.

2.1 AAL Technologies and Systems

The term Ambient Assisted Living (AAL) includes all assisting technologies or systems which contribute to the maintenance of autonomy in everyday life and are in particular applied in care for prevention and rehabilitation [14, 17]. AAL technologies cover a broad range of functions and applications reaching from monitoring of vital parameters and detection of falls or positions to reminders and smart home functionalities. Here, some prototypical examples are described. As a first example, Radio Frequency Identification (RFID) tags are frequently used in the area of (outdoor) tracking and detection of positions [18]. Further, integrating common Information and Communication Technologies (ICT) (e.g., movement sensors, (infra-red) cameras, microphones) into people's living environments enables different types of monitoring.

Those monitoring solutions aim for enhancing safety by detection of falls and emergencies in private home environments [19] as well as in professional care contexts such as hospitals or care institutions [20]. Besides those safety-relevant functions and safety-enhancing reasons, other types of AAL technologies aim for facilitating everyday life by using automated technologies such as memory aids or home automation [21, 22]. Further, another aim of AAL is the support of communication with families, friends, and caregivers by integrating ICT in home environments [14]. Wearable technologies (e.g., an emergency arm strap) represent a further area of AAL technologies and are worn on the body or integrated in clothes that are able to communicate with intelligent AAL systems or smart home environments [10, 23]. Along with those examples, numerous systems and technologies are available on the market [e.g., 24, 25] or focused in current research projects (e.g., [26]). However, those technologies and systems have not reached sustainable success of those systems so far, as they are only rarely used in real life [16] and in particular in professional care contexts [27].

This poses the question for what reasons the existing and assisting technologies (including their facilitating and supporting potential in everyday care contexts) are not widely used in professional care contexts? As future users' acceptance as well as their perception of benefits and barriers are decisive for a successful integration of AAL systems in everyday life, it is of major importance to understand the barriers of AAL usage in professional contexts. In this study, we therefore focused on professional caregivers as potential and important user group of these systems, their perceptions, ideas, wishes, and willingness to adopt home-integrated ICT.

2.2 Acceptance of AAL and the Diversity of Users

Previous research in the field of AAL technology acceptance revealed that AAL technologies were mostly evaluated positively and that in particular the necessity and usefulness of technical support were recognized as relevant benefits by diverse groups of potential users [26, 28–30]. In more detail, participants acknowledged the potential of AAL technologies to enable an independent and more autonomous life as well as a longer staying at the own home for older, diseased and/or disabled people. In contrast to perceived benefits, feelings of isolation [27, 31], feelings of surveillance, and invasion of privacy [32–34] were reported to be the most relevant barriers of AAL technology usage when the participants were asked to think about a concrete integration of those technologies in their living environment.

Previous qualitative research focused on people aged above 60 and their perceptions of AAL technologies in focus group [35, 36] and interview studies [30]: those studies revealed in accordance to the previously mentioned general positive perception, that older participants acknowledged the benefits of staying longer at the own home, understood the chances and potential of AAL technologies as well as the problematic lack of care staff. In contrast, the older participants expressed fears concerning a lack of personal contact referring to the concern that care staff will might be substituted by technologies, privacy concerns, and a dependency on technologies they are not able to control. Numerous quantitative surveys confirmed these mostly qualitative gained results (e.g., [29]).

So far, acceptance research has hardly considered the perspectives of professional care givers on integrating AAL technologies in professional care contexts, although their perspectives are mandatory in order to do justice to needs of care and care itself in professional care environments. Nevertheless, single studies have already focused on caregivers as potential users and on their perceived concerns regarding in-home monitoring technologies [37]. Further, other studies investigated the effectiveness of different technologies, analyzed requirements and the perception of AAL technology usage, and derived guidelines for design and implementation of AAL technologies in the context of professional care environments [38, 39].

Although the majority of studies in this regard revealed a general positive attitude towards AAL technologies, a conducted comparative study found a more attitude of professional caregivers towards AAL technologies compared to other user groups (people with disabilities, relatives of people with disabilities, and "not"-experienced people (neither professional expertise nor personal consternation)) [28]. These study results provided the basis searching for an explanation why AAL technologies are not widely used in professional care contexts and showed the importance to investigate the perceptions, wishes, and needs of professional caregivers as specific user group in depth. To fully understand the emerging negative attitude of professional caregivers it is important to analyze relevant acknowledged benefits and existing perceived barriers, specific data and technology configurations as well as their handling with regard to the specific user group and their specific usage contexts and situations.

In the past years, well-known acceptance models such as TAM and UTAUT as well as their adapted versions were urgently used to investigate the acceptance of assisting ICT and AAL technologies. Within the specific context of care and in light of increasing usage requirements in the context of care, the existing technology acceptance models are not sufficient due to (1) the sensible usage context of care, (2) the models' view of acceptance as static technology assessment, and (3) because of leaving apart trade-offs between simultaneously existing benefits and barriers and in particular analyses regarding user factor influences [40].

Therefore, we used interviews in a first step – specifically tailored to professional caregivers –in order to identify challenges in care focusing on perceived benefits as well as perceived barriers of AAL technology usage. Afterwards, we aimed for an identification of which technologies are exactly (not) allowed to be used by professional caregivers. For this purpose, we took the results from the preceding interview study and conceptualized an online questionnaire tailored to professional caregivers needs and wishes ensuring that all relevant aspects (for this specific user group) can be quantified.

3   Methodology

This section presents the methodological research design starting with the aim of the study, the procedure, and specific research questions. Afterwards, the empirical design of the quantitative online questionnaire study and the sample's characteristics are described.

3.1   Aim, Procedure, and Research Questions

Our study aimed for an investigation of professional caregivers' perception and acceptance of AAL technologies in professional care contexts. Thereby, perception referred to diverse dimensions (e.g., perception of potential benefits and barriers of AAL technology usage) with a potential to influence the acceptance operationalized as intention to use AAL technologies and systems (see Fig. 1). In more detail, the study aimed for answers to the following research questions. including the following research questions:

- How do professional caregivers evaluate specific staff- and patient related benefits and barriers of using AAL technologies? (RQ 1)
- How should data handling be realized? In more detail: Which data is allowed to be gathered, which technologies should be used to gather data, and how are data access and storage duration evaluated by professional caregivers? (RQ 2)
- Do relationships between user factors and the acceptance and perception of AAL technologies exist? (RQ 3)
- Are there significant influences of user factors on the perception of AAL technologies? (RQ4)
- Which factors are most decisive for AAL technology acceptance? (RQ5)
- Do those factors differ for diverse user groups based on demographic and attitudinal characteristics? (RQ6)

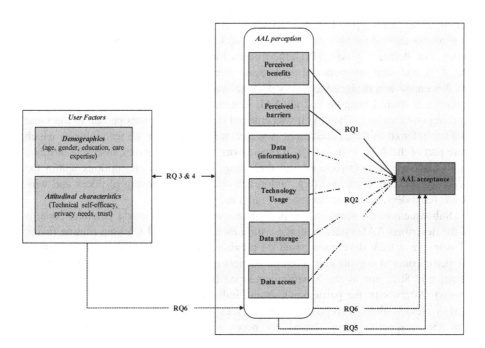

Fig. 1. Research model and research questions.

In accordance with the research questions and model (Fig. 1), we were in a first step interested in identifying probably relevant perceived staff- and patient-related benefits and barriers of AAL technology usage (RQ1) in professional care contexts. Afterwards, it was of importance to analyze the way in which handling of data/information should be realized in professional care contexts (RQ2). For this purpose, it was necessary to ask professional caregivers specifically for their opinions and respectively evaluations of diverse types of data allowed to be gathered, specific technologies allowed to be used to gather data as well as to what extent data is allowed to be stored or be accessible for third persons. Based on these fundamental evaluations, it was possible to investigate potential relationships between user factors and the perception and acceptance of AAL technologies (RQ3). Subsequently, identified relationships could be used as indicators for analyzing significant influences of user factors on the acceptance and perception of AAL technologies (RQ4). Finally, it was of importance to analyze which of the relevant and influencing factors is most decisive for AAL technology acceptance (RQ5). Besides insights for the whole group of participants, it had to be investigated if different factors are most decisive for diverse groups of professional caregivers (RQ6).

3.2 Empirical Design of Online Questionnaire

Findings of previous interview studies provided the basis for the conceptualization of the questionnaire including the development of questionnaire items. The first part of the questionnaire contained queries of demographic characteristics such as age, gender, education, duration of professional experience, and care sector (i.e. geriatric care, nursing care, care/support of disabled people). Afterwards, the participants were asked to evaluate individual attitudinal characteristics, namely their technical self-efficacy (using four items, $\alpha = .884$; [41]), their needs for privacy (using six items, $\alpha = .833$; [42, 43]), and their interpersonal trust (using three items, $\alpha = .793$ [44]).

A scenario was designed as a very personal everyday working situation wherein the participants should imagine that an AAL system was integrated in their professional working environment. Thereby, it was ensured that all participants pertain to the same baseline referred to the evaluation of AAL technology. Further, all technologies which were part of the AAL system (e.g., room sensors, ultrasonic sensors, microphones, and video cameras) were introduced and their range of functions and options within the AAL system were explained (e.g., automatic opening and closing of doors and windows, reminders, alarms (emergencies, falls) etc.).

Subsequent to the scenario, the participants were asked to assess potential benefits of the described AAL system's usage within their professional working routine (using 14 items, $\alpha = .923$; developed based on previous interview studies' results). Further, the participants also evaluated potential barriers of the AAL system's usage (using 17 items; $\alpha = .861$; just as the benefits developed based on previous interview studies' results). Afterwards, the participants should indicate whether – in their opinion – the AAL system is allowed to gather different types of data (using 14 items (data types), $\alpha = .856$; respective items based on necessary information to realize technical functions).

In accordance with the data types, the participants were asked to evaluate different technologies' usage to gather data (using 12 items, $\alpha = .892$; based on technical configurations of AAL systems). To evaluate the acceptance of the AAL system, the participants evaluated six different statements ($\alpha = .932$) dealing with their general perception of the system (e.g., "I find the described AAL system useful") as well as an concrete intention to use the system. During the assessment, all described items had to be evaluated on six-point Likert scales (1 = min: "I strongly disagree"; 6 = max: "I strongly agree") and are presented in the results section.

At the end of the questionnaire, the participants were given opportunity to reason their opinions on an optional basis and to provide their feedback concerning the study. On average, the participants needed 20 min to complete the questionnaire. Data was collected online in Germany and the questionnaire was made available for 3 months in spring and summer 2017. Participants were recruited in online networks as well as by personal and project contact to care institutions.

3.3 Participants and User Factor Segmentation

Overall, a total of 287 participants volunteered to participate in our questionnaire study. As only complete data sets and suitable data sets (filled out by professional care givers) could be used for statistical analyses, 113 data sets had to be excluded and a sample of n = 174 remained. Most of the professional caregivers were acquired by personal and by direct contact to professional care institutions. The mean age of the participants was on average 36.3 years ($SD = 11.2$; $min = 19$; $max = 68$) and the participants were predominantly female (74.7%) (25.3% male). The majority of the participants indicated a completed apprenticeship (42.5%) as their highest educational level, while each 23.0% reported to hold a university degree and a university entrance diploma. Further, 7.5% indicated to hold a secondary school certificate, while 4.0% reported other certificates.

All of the participants worked or have worked as professional caregivers: the majority of them (52.9%, n = 92) in the area of care and support of people with disabilities, while 25.9% (n = 45) worked in the area geriatric and 21.3% (n = 37) in nursing care. On average, the caregivers indicated to be long-term experienced in professional care: 43.5% (n = 74) reported to have more than 10 years care expertise, 41.8% (n = 71) between 3 and 10 years, and only 14.7% (n = 25) indicated to have less than 3 years professional experience.

With regard to attitudinal variables, the participants reported to have on average a middle technical self-efficacy (TSE) ($M = 3.4$; $SD = 0.7$; $min = 1$; $max = 6$) and also a middle interpersonal trust ($M = 3.5$; $SD = 0.8$; $min = 1$; $max = 6$). The participants' needs for privacy and data security were on average rather high ($M = 4.2$; $SD = 0.9$; $min = 1$; $max = 6$).

For detailed analyses referring to potential influences of user factors on the perception and acceptance of AAL technologies it was necessary to segment specific user groups based on the respective frequency distribution and content-related fit. For *age*, it was decided to distinguish between "younger" participants aged under 40 years (63.5%) and "older" participants aged 40 years and older (36.5%). For *care expertise*, it was tried to compared short- and long-term experience by dividing the participants in two groups: "beginners" with less than 10 years professional care experience and "old stagers" having more than 10 years professional care experience. For both attitudinal variables, the mean of the scale (3.5) was used as group cut-off. Regarding technical self-efficacy this cut-off resulted in a group with a "low TSE" (62.5%) and a group with a "high TSE" (37.5%). Considering privacy needs, the segmentation revealed a smaller group with a "low privacy need" (26.5%) and a larger group with a "high privacy need" (73.5%).

4   Results

Before descriptive and inference analyses were conducted, item analyses were calculated to ensure measurement quality, while a Cronbach's alpha >0.7 indicated a satisfying internal consistency of the scales. Data was analyzed descriptively, and in addition we used inferential statistics to identify user diversity effects, by correlation, (M)ANOVA, and linear regression analysis. The level of significance was set at 5%.

Based on a preceding study [45], the results were first presented descriptively for the perception of benefits and barriers identifying decisive factors for the acceptance of AAL. Thereby, (a) staff- and patient-related benefits and barriers, (b) data gathering and applied technologies, as well as (c) data access and storage duration are illuminated. In a second step, it is analyzed whether and to which extent user factors (e.g., professional care experience, needs for privacy) impact the perception of AAL. In a last step, it is investigated which factors are most decisive for AAL acceptance differing between (a) the whole sample of the participants and (b) specific user groups among the participants.

4.1   Perception of AAL Technologies

This section presents the results concerning the perception of benefits and barriers of using AAL systems in professional care contexts (RQ1). Further, it is investigated which data is allowed to be gathered, how the data should be gathered, who should have access to the data, and for how long data access should be allowed. Thereby, the results initially refer to the whole sample of caregivers investigating (RQ 2).

Perception of Staff- and Patient-Related Benefits and Barriers. Figure 2 presents the evaluation of perceived staff- (left side) and patient-related (right side) **benefits** of an AAL system's usage. Among the staff-related benefits, *fast Assistance in emergencies* ($M = 4.6$; $SD = 1.2$) was perceived as the most important benefit, followed by a *higher control in everyday working life* ($M = 4.0$; $SD = 1.5$), *relief in documentation of care* ($M = 3.9$; $SD = 1.4$), *simplified proof of rendered care* ($M = 3.9$; $SD = 1.4$), *relief in everyday working life* ($M = 3.8$; $SD = 1.4$), and *time savings in everyday working life* ($M = 3.7$; $SD = 1.3$), which were all rated only slightly positively. An *increase of working quality* ($M = 3.5$; $SD = 1.4$) was evaluated neutrally and was thus not seen as a relevant benefit of using AAL systems. In contrast, the two aspects *lower fear to be able to do own mistakes* ($M = 2.9$; $SD = 1.5$) and *measure against crisis in care* ($M = 2.9$; $SD = 1.6$) were evaluated slightly negatively and were thus rejected to be benefits of AAL technologies in professional care contexts. Among the patient-related benefits, *increase in safety* (M = 4.3; SD = 1.2) represented the most important aspect. In comparison, other potential benefits such as *relief in everyday life* (M = 3.8 SD = 1.3), *extension of autonomy* (M = 3.7; SD = 1.4), or *reduction of dependency* (M = 3.5; SD = 1.4) were rated only slightly positively or almost neutrally.

In contrast to a comparatively diverse evaluation of benefits revealing accepted ("real") and rejected potential benefits, none of the potential **barriers** was rejected (see Fig. 3). Strong agreements of almost all potential barriers of using AAL systems showed that nearly all aspects were perceived as solid, "real" barriers of AAL technology usage in professional care contexts. In particular, aspects dealing with privacy and data security (e.g., *invasion in privacy* (M = 5.2; SD = 1.0), *data abuse by third parties* (M = 4.8; SD = 1.2), *recording of data* (M = 4.7; SD = 1.3)) as well as with a perceived surveillance (i.e. *surveillance by technology* (M = 5.0; SD = 1.1), *control by supervisors* (M = 4.9; SD = 1.2), *control by colleagues* (M = 4.6; SD = 1.3)) were rated highest and represent relevant barriers of AAL technology usage in professional care contexts.

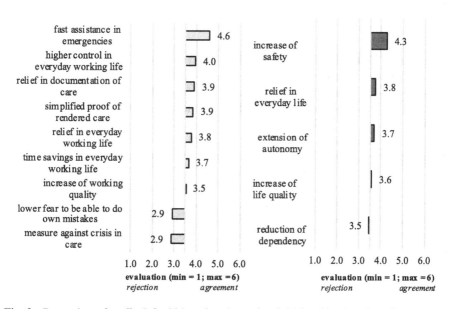

Fig. 2. Perception of staff- (left side) and patient-related (right side) benefits of using AAL technologies and systems.

Fear of isolation (M = 4.1; SD = 1.4), *missing trust in technical functionality* (M = 3.9; SD = 1.4), or *interruption of routines* (M = 3.9; SD = 1.3) were evaluated slightly positively and were thus slightly confirmed to be barriers of AAL technology usage. In contrast, *handling seems to be too complex* (M = 3.5; SD = 1.3) and *confrontation with new technology* (M = 3.4; SD = 1.4) were rated neutrally and thus, those aspects do not represent notably relevant barriers of AAL technology usage.

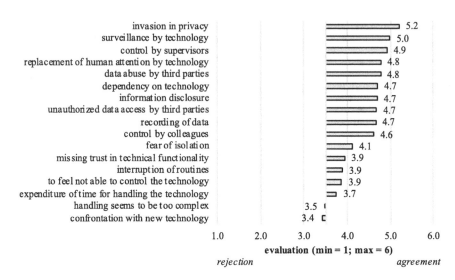

Fig. 3. Perception of potential barriers of AAL technology usage in professional care contexts (based on [45]).

Realization of Data Handling: What, How, for How Long, and for Whom? The participants were also asked for their perception of data handling with regard to AAL technologies (RQ2). Thereby, the participants evaluated which data should be allowed to be gathered and which specific technology should be used to gather data.

With regard to **data allowed to be gathered** (see Fig. 4) it was striking that gathering of information related with emergency situations (*emergencies (falls epileptic seizures)* ($M = 5.3$; $SD = 0.9$), *actuation of emergency buttons* (*care staff*: $M = 5.2$; $SD = 1.0$; *inhabitants*: $M = 5.2$; $SD = 1.0$), and *cries for help/support* $M = 5.2$; $SD = 1.0$) was clearly accepted. To gather patient-related information was partly evaluated slightly positively, e.g., about *fixations* ($M = 4.1$; $SD = 1.6$) and *rooms (opening windows, doors, ...)* ($M = 4.0$; $SD = 1.6$). Otherwise, gathering the *patients' position* ($M = 3.6$; $SD = 1.4$) was evaluated neutrally, while gathering data about *sleeping* ($M = 3.3$; $SD = 1.5$) was slightly rejected. Interestingly, to gather the *position of care staff* ($M = 2.8$; $SD = 1.5$) was clearly evaluated more negatively than gathering the patients' position.

Considering care-related information, a clear rejecting pattern is striking: to gather information about the *duration of care* ($M = 3.0$; $SD = 1.6$), *whole care situations* ($M = 2.9$; $SD = 1.6$), and *times (rooms are entered or left)* ($M = 2.9$; $SD = 1.5$) was slightly rejected, while gathering data concerning a *24 h observation* ($M = 2.6$; $SD = 1.6$) and *talks during care* ($M = 2.1$; $SD = 1.4$) was clearly rated negatively and was thus not accepted.

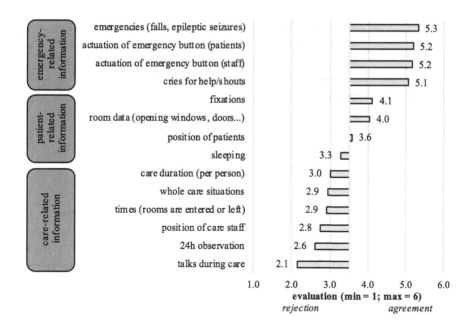

Fig. 4. Evaluation of data (information) allowed to be gathered in professional care contexts (based on [45]).

In accordance with the diverse evaluation of the type of gathered data, the specific **technologies** that are allowed to be used to gather data were also evaluated quite differently (Fig. 5). Consistent with the evaluation of emergency-related information, using *emergency buttons* (*patients: M* = 5.1; *SD* = 1.1; *staff: M* = 5.1; *SD* = 1.2) and *fall sensors into the floor* (*M* = 4.8; *SD* = 1.4) was clearly accepted. In addition, *fall sensors in clothes on body of patients* (*M* = 4.3; *SD* = 1.5) and *room sensors* (*M* = 4.1; *SD* = 1.6) were rated positively. Usage of *motion detectors* (*in rooms: M* = 3.4; *SD* = 1.6; *in clothes of patients: M* = 3.3; *SD* = 1.6) as well as *ultrasonic sensors* (*M* = 3.3; *SD* = 1.5) was marginally rejected.

In contrast, *infra-red cameras* (*M* = 2.5; *SD* = 1.4), *motion detectors in clothes of staff* (*M* = 2.5; *SD* = 1.5), *microphones* (*M* = 2.4; *SD* = 1.4), and *cameras* (*M* = 2.2; *SD* = 1.3) were evaluated clearly negatively and were thus not accepted to be used to gather data in professional care contexts.

Besides the evaluation of specific information and technologies, the participants further assessed the storage duration and data access (Fig. 6).

Concerning **data access**, the most positive evaluations were found for *room data:* it was evaluated slightly positively (or at least tolerated) to be accessible for colleagues (*M* = 4.0; *SD* = 1.6), direct supervisors (*M* = 3.9; *SD* = 1.6), and all supervisors (*M* = 3.7; *SD* = 1.7). Conversely, negative evaluations showed that *position data, audio data,* and *video data* should neither be accessible for all supervisors (*position: M* = 2.4; *SD* = 1.5, *audio: M* = 2.0; *SD* = 1.4, *video: M* = 2.2; *SD* = 1.4), direct supervisors (*position: M* = 2.8; *SD* = 1.6, *audio: M* = 2.5; *SD* = 1.6, *video: M* = 2.7; *SD* = 1.6), nor colleagues (*position: M* = 2.9; *SD* = 1.6, *audio: M* = 2.3; *SD* = 1.5, *video: M* = 2.6; *SD* = 1.5).

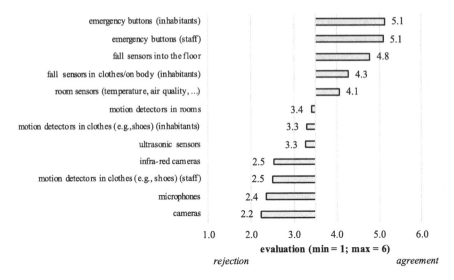

Fig. 5. Evaluation of technologies allowed for data gathering in professional care contexts [45].

With regard to the evaluation of **storage duration,** comparably positive values showed that data should *only be allowed to be evaluated for the moment* independent from the data type (*room: M* = 4.1; *SD* = 1.5; *position: M* = 4.0; *SD* = 1.6; *video: M* = 3.8; *SD* = 1.7; *audio: M* = 3.8; *SD* = 1.8). *Data storage on a daily basis* (*position: M* = 2.8; *SD* = 1.5; *audio: M* = 2.6; *SD* = 1.6; *video: M* = 2.6; *SD* = 1.5) and in particular *long-term storage* (*position: M* = 2.1; *SD* = 1.3; *audio: M* = 1.8; *SD* = 1.1; *video: M* = 1.9; *SD* = 1.2) were partly clearly rejected for all data types except of *room data. Room data* was evaluated almost neutrally for *storage on a daily basis* (*M* = 3.7; *SD* = 1.7) as well as *long-term storage* (*M* = 3.4; *SD* = 1.8) indicating that data storage was most likely tolerated with regard to *room data.*

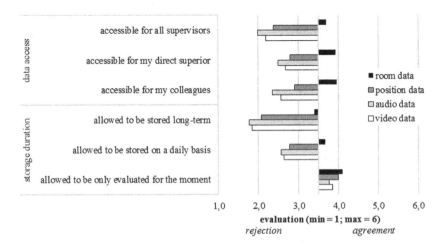

Fig. 6. Perception of data access and data storage for different data types (based on [45]).

4.2   Do User Factors Influence Professional Caregivers' Perception of AAL?

So far, predominantly descriptive results referring to the whole sample of caregivers have been presented. Now, the results are analyzed in more detail focusing on potential influences of demographic and attitudinal characteristics on the perception and acceptance of AAL technologies. For this purpose, correlation analyses were conducted in a first step to find out which demographic and attitudinal characteristics are possibly relevant for the acceptance of AAL technologies (Fig. 7).

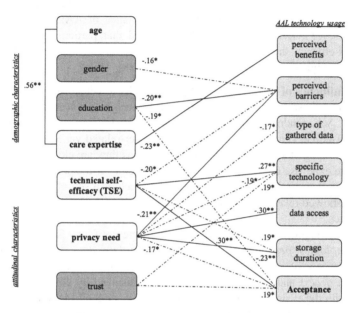

Fig. 7. Correlations between user factors and the evaluation of AAL technologies (adapted from [45]).

Relationships Between User Factors and AAL Perception (RQ3). Considering demographic characteristics, the results revealed single correlations with regard to the perception and acceptance of AAL technology usage. First, it was striking that age was not related at all with one of the perception and acceptance dimensions. Instead, it correlated strongly with the participant's duration of care expertise ($\rho = .564; p < .01$). In turn, the duration of care expertise was the own variable which was related with the perception of benefits ($\rho = -.233; p < .01$). Further, gender exclusively correlated only slightly with the perceived barriers of AAL technology usage ($\rho = -.156; p < .05$) revealing that women showed a slightly higher evaluation of perceived barriers than men. Education was slightly related with the perception of barriers ($\rho = -.202; p < .01$) and the acceptance of AAL technologies ($\rho = .196; p < .05$).

More striking relationships were found with regard to attitudinal characteristics. For interpersonal trust, there were indeed only slight single correlations with the evaluation of specific technologies ($\rho = .189$; $p < .05$) and acceptance of AAL technologies ($\rho = .186$; $p < .05$). In contrast, the results showed stronger correlations for the two attitudinal variables privacy need and technical self-efficacy (TSE). The analysis revealed strongest correlations for the participants' privacy need and the perception of barriers ($\rho = .209$; $p < .01$), data access ($\rho = -.301$; $p < .01$), and storage duration ($\rho = -.228$; $p < .01$). Those correlations indicated that participants with higher needs for privacy showed higher evaluations of perceived barriers and a more negative attitude towards data access and long-term data storage. Referring to the technical self-efficacy of the participants, the strongest relationships were found for the evaluation of specific technologies ($\rho = .274$; $p < .01$) and acceptance of AAL technology usage ($\rho = .299$; $p < .01$). Here, the correlations indicated that participants with a higher technical self-efficacy showed a more positive attitude towards specific applied technologies and a higher acceptance of AAL technologies.

Significant Influence of User Factors (RQ4). In order to get a broader understanding of the influence of user factors on professional care personnel's acceptance of assistive technologies, we conducted MANOVA analyses **including age, care expertise, technical self-efficacy,** and **needs for privacy** as user-related variables. Age and care expertise were integrated in the MANOVA analyses as they are closely related to each other and care expertise seems to be an explaining factor for the perception of benefits. The attitudinal characteristics need for privacy and technical self-efficacy were chosen as they each showed relationships to several dimensions of AAL technology perception and acceptance.

Interestingly, significant effects of user factors were not found for the evaluation of *specific technologies, permitted gathering of specific data, data storage, data access,* and the *acceptance of assistive technologies.* In contrast, the evaluation of *perceived benefits, data access* and *perceived barriers* was influenced by different user factors.

Starting with the evaluation of benefits, significant overall effects were found for **age** ($F(14, 123) = 1.947$; $p < .05$) and **professional care expertise** ($F(1, 123) = 1.866$; $p < .05$). Referring to **age**, specifically the benefit of a higher control in the everyday working life ($F(1, 151) = 4.545$; $p < .05$) was evaluated significantly more positively by younger care professionals aged under 40 years ($M = 4.1$; $SD = 1.5$) compared to older care professionals ($M = 3.6$; $SD = 1.4$).

With regard to **professional care expertise,** the pattern was found that professional "beginners" (less than 10 years professional experience) evaluated some of the perceived benefits significantly more positively than professional "old stagers" (more than 10 years professional experience). In more detail (see Fig. 8), professional "beginners" acknowledged the benefits *simplified proof of rendered care* ($F(1, 151) = 11.515$; $p < .01$), *relief in everyday life* (for their "patients") ($F(1, 151) = 5.051$; $p < .05$) and *time savings in everyday working life* ($F(1, 151) = 4.444$; $p < .05$) more than the "old stagers". Further, the benefit of an *increase of working quality* ($F(1, 151) = 4.680$;

p < .05) was evaluated slightly positively by the "beginners", while it was slightly rejected by the "old stagers". Finally, "old stagers" rejected the benefits of a potential *measure against crisis in care* ($F(1, 151) = 4.969$; $p < .05$) and the *lower fear to be able to do own mistakes* ($F(1, 151) = 5.957$; $p < .05$) more strongly than the professional "beginners".

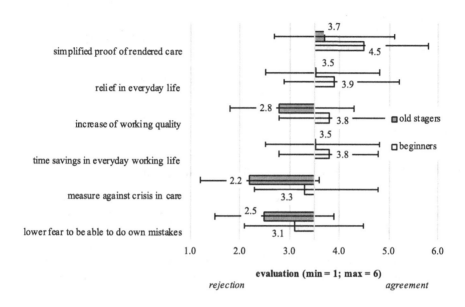

Fig. 8. Significant differences between professional "beginners" and "old stagers" regarding the perception of perceived benefits.

With regard to the perception of barriers, significant influences of user factors were neither found for **age** nor for **professional expertise**. In contrast, individual needs for privacy influenced the perception of barriers significantly ($F(17, 124) = 1.777$; $p < .05$). In more detail (see Fig. 9), people with a high privacy need confirmed the potential barriers of *invasion in privacy* ($F(1, 151) = 4.921$; $p < .05$), *unauthorized data access by third parties* ($F(1, 151) = 5.586$; $p < .05$), and *replacement of human attention* by technology ($F(1, 151) = 4.053$; $p < .05$) significantly more than participants with a low privacy need. This pattern occurred even more with regard to the barriers *surveillance by technology* ($F(1, 151) = 2.823$; $p < .01$) and *data abuse by third parties* ($F(1, 151) = 11.187$; $p < .01$) showing a significantly stronger agreement of participants with a high privacy need compared to people with a low privacy need.

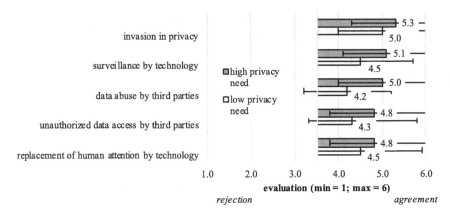

Fig. 9. Significant differences between participants with a high and a low privacy needs regarding the perception of barriers.

4.3 What Is the Most Decisive Factor for AAL Acceptance?

The descriptive results showed that the acceptance of the mentioned AAL technologies was overall evaluated rather neutrally (M = 3.6; SD = 1.3), while comparatively *a system consisting only of room sensors* (M = 4.0; SD = 1.5) received the highest and a *system consisting of all mentioned technologies except of a camera* was (M = 2.9; SD = 1.4) the lowest evaluations. In order to analyze, which of the descriptively as well as inference statistically analyzed and presented factors influences the acceptance of AAL technologies the most, a step-wise linear regression analysis was conducted. In a first step, this analysis referred to all participants. Afterwards, the analysis procedure was conducted for diverse user groups.

Most Decisive Factors for the Whole Sample (RQ5). Within the regression analyses, the acceptance of AAL technology usage was calculated as dependent variable, while perceived benefits, perceived barriers, data that is allowed to be gathered, specific type of technology, data access, and storage duration represented the independent variables. The calculation revealed four significant models: The first model predicted 59.1% (adj. r^2 = .591) variance of AAL technology acceptance based on the *specific technology* that is used to gather data. The second model additionally contained *perceived benefits* and explained +8.5% (adj. r^2 = .676) variance of AAL technology acceptance. The third model explained +3.2% (adj. r^2 = .708) variance based on the specific technology, perceived benefits, and additionally on the *type of gathered data*. The fourth and final model explained +2.2% (adj. r^2 = .730) variance of AAL technology acceptance and contained besides perceived benefits, specific technology, type of gathered data, also *perceived barriers*. Interestingly, the other two integrated dimensions *data access* and *storage duration* were not part of the regression models. Thus, those dimensions did not influence the acceptance of AAL technologies significantly. Figure 10 illustrates the final regression model and displays the regression coefficient β for all independent variables.

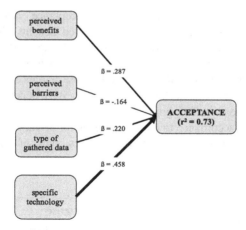

Fig. 10. Final regression model for all participants based on significantly influencing variables [45].

Explaining Acceptance for Diverse User Groups (RQ6). Each two demographic (*age* and *care expertise*) and attitudinal variables (*technical self-efficacy* and *privacy need*) were integrated as user group variables into the regression analyses. (Figure 11).

Starting with the *age groups*, the final regression model for "younger" care persons aged under 40 years explained 72.8% variance of AAL acceptance based on the perception and evaluation of the technology used to gather data, the type of gathered data, and benefits of AAL technology usage. For "older" care professionals (aged 40 and older), the final regression model reached a slightly higher proportion of explained variance of AAL acceptance ($r^2 = .739$) and of the type of technology used to gather data and perceived benefits of AAL technology usage. In contrast to the "younger" participants' model, the "older" participants' model based additionally on perceived barriers of AAL technology usage.

Referring to the *care expertise groups* a very similar pattern can be observed: the final regression model for care "beginners" (less than 10 years professional care expertise) explained 71.1% variance of AAL technology acceptance and based in accordance with the "younger" group of participants on the evaluations of the technology used to gather data, the type of gathered data, and benefits of AAL technology usage. In contrast, the final regression model for the "old stagers" (having more than 10 years professional care expertise) explained a higher proportion of AAL acceptance' variance ($r^2 = .786$) and based on the specific technologies and benefits of AAL technology usage. In accordance with the "older" group of the participants, the "old stagers" model additionally based on the perception of barriers of AAL technology usage.

In addition, regression analyses were also conducted for the attitudinal variables privacy needs and TSE. Starting with *privacy needs* (Fig. 11), the final model for participants with "low privacy needs" explained 61.4% variance of AAL acceptance based on the evaluation of specific technologies and perceived benefits of AAL technology usage. Conversely, the final regression model for participants with "high needs for privacy" explained a higher proportion of AAL acceptance' variance ($r^2 = .766$) of and based besides specific technologies and perceived benefits also on the type of gathered data as well as perceived barriers of AAL technology usage.

A similar pattern is observed for the two *technical self-efficacy (TSE:* the regression model for people with a "high TSE" explained 73.4% variance of AAL acceptance based on the dimensions used technology and perceived benefits. In contrast, the regression model for the "low TSE group" reached 70.6% variance of AAL technology acceptance, based – in accordance to the "high needs for privacy" group – on the four dimensions: specific technologies, perceived barriers, type of data, and perceived benefits.

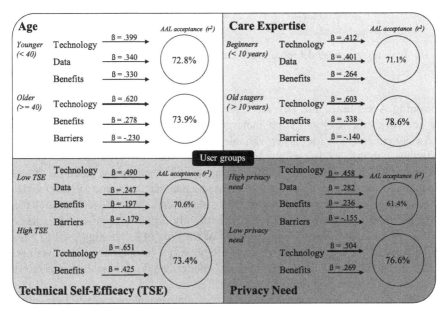

Fig. 11. Results of regression analyses referring to different user groups: age, care expertise, TSE, and privacy needs.

5   Discussion

The present study aimed for a better understanding of (a) professional caregivers' perspectives on the acceptance of specific AAL technologies in professional care environments as well as (b) the influence of professional caregivers' individual factors on technology acceptance. We aimed for a detailed analysis of the requirements and wishes of this specific stakeholder group, as professional caregivers play a decisive role for the acceptance of AAL technologies in professional care environments. This study's results provide valuable insights into acceptance-decisive factors of AAL technologies in professional care contexts (see Sect. 5.1) and should be taken into account for the development, design, and configuration of AAL technologies. Further, the results showed that professional caregivers' acceptance and perception of AAL technologies is influenced by individual factors (e.g., age, care expertise, privacy needs) (see Sect. 5.2).

5.1 Acceptance of AAL Technologies and Systems (*RQ 1 & 2 & 5*)

The professional caregivers' evaluations of perceived benefits, perceived barriers, and AAL technology acceptance (see RQ 1) differ clearly from previous findings with regard to AAL technology acceptance. In contrast to a general positive evaluation of AAL technologies that has been found in numerous past studies (e.g., [26, 30]), professional caregivers – we consulted in this study – expressed a very restrained and critical attitude towards AAL technologies and showed, if at all, neutral acceptance evaluations. Confirming a preceding study [28], this study verifies that professional caregivers are much more critical with regard to the integration of assisting technologies in their professional everyday life than other user groups. This is indicated by two different patterns:

First, it was striking that the participants showed only low agreements of potential benefits. Except of benefits that deal with a faster assistance in emergencies, all benefits are evaluated only with rather positive or rather negative i.e. primarily neutral values. Therefore, some potential benefits (e.g., measure against care crisis) are not even perceived as real benefits. This phenomenon can maybe be explained by the applied methodology of the scenario-based approach: previous studies have already proven that hands-on experience with AAL technologies has the potential to lead to more positive perceptions of usage motives [33]. Hence, it can be expected that professional caregivers would also evaluate AAL technologies differently if they would have the chance to try and test those technologies in their professional everyday life.

Otherwise, the more negative and critical attitude of professional caregivers is expressed by comparably unknown, high agreements of barriers: with regard to the results it is striking that none of the potential barriers is rejected and this indicates, that all potential barriers are perceived as real barriers and severe drawbacks. These results clearly contradict previous research results which revealed a much lower reluctance to AAL systems and a lower confirmation of perceived barriers (e.g., [28, 34]). Our results showed that in particular the aspects of a potential invasion of privacy, data security concerns, and a feeling of surveillance represent the most relevant perceived barriers for professional caregivers. In this context, it is a noteworthy finding that the by professional caregivers perceived relevant barriers center around their own professional person. The most severe concern deals with the concern to be tracked or controlled. The patients or better the caretakers, for which caregivers are responsible and which could seriously profit from AAL systems, are not taken into account when thinking about barriers of using AAL technologies.

Also, the perception and evaluation of specific data and technology configurations are decisive for the AAL technology acceptance (RQ 5). In more detail, the study revealed insights into the perceptions of professional caregivers referring to which specific data should be allowed to be gathered and which specific technology should be used to gather data, if at all (RQ 2). The results show clearly that – from the perspective of professional caregivers – only emergency-related data is allowed to be gathered.

Gathering of all other data types is rejected or, if at all, just tolerated. This evaluation pattern significantly contradicts the functions caregivers want AAL technologies to undertake: i.e. the participants reported in open comment fields and interviews that e.g., in some cases detection of positions of care staff and patients is useful and desirable, for which gathering different data types is factually necessary. In accordance with the evaluation of specific data configuration, the evaluation of specific technologies that should be used for data collection shows similar results: the professional caregivers indicate to accept solely technologies that are partly already existing (e.g., emergency buttons) or gather only static, binary data (e.g., room sensors). However, the caregivers rejected more complex technologies with a potential higher privacy invasion (e.g., cameras, microphones). These results are in line with previous research results (e.g., [29]) and illustrate the opposition between the desired technical functionality (that could support professional caregivers in caring) and the admitted specific data and technology configurations. The evaluation of data storage and data access completes the professional caregivers' negative attitude and evaluation of perceived barriers: the professional caregivers do not want that data is accessible to colleagues or supervisors and data should only be processed - not stored. As data is not needed to be stored long-term for most of the functions AAL technologies could undertake, targeted communication strategies should focus on handling of data (e.g., only processing, not storage) and could this way may help to dismantle perceived barriers and especially caveats concerning privacy and data security.

5.2 Diversity of Users Matters (*RQ 3 & 4 & 6*)

The in a first step correlation analysis based integration of user diversity factors into the analysis of AAL technology acceptance shows that most of the demographic characteristics of the professional caregivers are not decisive and do not influence the caregivers' acceptance of AAL technologies (see RQ 3). The own demographic aspect revealing a significant relationship to the perception of AAL technologies, in specific the evaluation of benefits. Additionally, the analysis revealed that – not surprisingly – the participants age is related with their professional care experience. In contrast, the results suggested that attitudinal characteristics are more relevant and influence the perception of AAL technologies (e.g., TSE, privacy needs). These correlation analysis results enabled and initiated deeper analyses of the variables age related with care expertise, TSE, and privacy needs (RQ4 and RQ6).

As a new and so far unexplored relationship, the results revealed care expertise as the only factor explaining differences in the perception of benefits regarding the usage of AAL technologies: younger care professionals with less care expertise had a much more open attitude towards AAL technologies applied in professional care contexts expressed by significantly higher evaluations of potential benefits of AAL technology usage. In contrast, older care professionals with longer care expertise showed a more restrained attitude and did not acknowledge the benefits of AAL technology usage. In accordance with this evaluation patterns, perceived benefits of AAL technology usage were part of the explaining regression model for AAL acceptance for the younger, less experienced care professionals, while perceived barriers were part of the explaining model for the older, more experienced care professionals.

Further, the results show that the participants technical self-efficacy (TSE) as well as their needs for privacy influence the acceptance and perceptions of AAL technologies significantly. In accordance with previous studies (e.g., [46]), the results revealed the evaluation pattern that people with a higher technical self-efficacy show a higher acceptance of AAL technologies mostly influenced by the type of technology and perceived benefits. In contrast, people with a lower technical self-efficacy have a more restrained attitude concerning the acceptance of AAL technology the evaluations of the type of technology and perceived benefits but additionally also the type of gathered data as well as perceived barriers.

A similar pattern was revealed for professional caregivers with different needs for privacy: people with low needs for privacy show a considerably higher AAL technology acceptance mostly influenced by type of technology and perceived benefits. In contrast, people with high needs for privacy have a lower acceptance, mostly influenced by type of technology, perceived benefits, perceived barriers, and type of data. In accordance with that, people with higher needs for privacy showed also stronger confirmations of barriers that dealt with privacy, surveillance, and data security.

To sum up, professional caregivers' age in relationship with their care expertise, their technical self-efficacy, and their need for privacy contribute to a different emphasis referring to the perception of benefits, barriers, and caveats (i.e. data gathering, storage, access, and privacy). This confirms (see Sect. 5.1) that especially the way AAL technologies handle data should be focused in future studies and should be integrated in communication referring to AAL technologies in professional environments.

5.3 Limitations and Future Research

This study provided valuable insights into AAL technology acceptance of professional caregivers in professional care contexts. In specific, it enables a better understanding of evaluations of specific benefits and barriers as well as concrete data and technology configurations. However, there are some limitations concerning the applied method and sample that should be considered in future approaches.

The present study was conceptualized as a first scenario-based approach focusing on professional caregivers' acceptance of AAL technologies, their perceptions of benefits and barriers as well as on their evaluations of technologies and data configurations. As mentioned before, the applied methodological approach was based on a scenario and thus, on a fictional and not on a real AAL system: this could probably influence the evaluations and may lead to an underestimation of potential benefits and an overestimation of potential barriers [33]. Thus, we aim for hands-on evaluations of AAL technologies in future studies focusing on professional caregivers and respectively usage of AAL technologies in professional care environments enabled by project contact and collaboration to care institutions.

A first aspect referring to the sample refers to the sample size as well as balance of demographic characteristics, which was sufficient - in particular, referred to the condition that only professional caregivers took part in the study. A higher proportion of female participants in the sample represents and fits to the higher proportion of women working in care institutions [47]. In addition, we are currently working on an investigation of potential care sector influences (geriatric care, nursing care, care of disabled people) on the acceptance and perception of AAL technologies in professional contexts due to different challenges and processes in the respective sectors.

Finally, this study focused German participants and therefore it represents the perspective of professional caregivers of one specific country with a specific background and in particular a specific health care system. From literature, we already know that the acceptance of AAL technologies differs with regard to different countries, their cultures and their specific healthcare systems. Hence, we aim for direct comparisons by conducting our approaches to be able to directly compare and analyze AAL acceptance depending on different countries, their backgrounds, and cultures.

6 Conclusion

This study focused on caregivers' perspectives on AAL technology usage in professional care contexts. Also, individual user factors, age and the professional expertise as well as the technical self-efficacy and the need for privacy with respect to the collected data during care were explored. The results reveal a critical perspective on digital care technologies out of the perspective of care personnel. The reasons for the negative attitude are not related to the usage of novel technology as such, but mostly to relevant concerns of loss of control, the fear of losing contact to the patients and, foremost, concerns about data collection and the unwished use of it by employers or care institutions. With increasing professional experience, the more reluctant if not deprecatory are attitudes towards care technologies. In addition, low technical competence and a high need of privacy aggravate the situation.

The findings are noteworthy if not alarming. As the increasing demographic change and the lack in the care supply necessitate new (technical) solutions, this situation needs urgently support by professional trainings, and a responsible policy which is reliable for care personnel. It is a mandatory claim, therefore, to (1) include care personnel's perspectives in defining sensible and appropriate care scenarios, in which technology has a well-balanced and harmonized role, to (2) develop novel technologies in line and with the help of experienced care personnel and to (3) inform care institutions and employers about this fragile and sensible perspective and to shape technology innovation in care institutions with care.

Acknowledgements. This work was partly funded by the German Federal Ministry of Education and Research projects Whistle (16SV7530) and PAAL (6SV7955).

References

1. Pickard, L.: A growing care gap? The supply of unpaid care for older people by their adult children in England to 2032. Ageing Soc. **35**(1), 96–123 (2015)
2. Walker, A., Maltby, T.: Active ageing: a strategic policy solution to demographic ageing in the European Union. Int. J. Soc. Welf. **21**, 117–130 (2012)

3. Bloom, D.E., Canning, D.: Global Demographic Change: Dimensions and Economic Significance National Bureau of Economic Research. Working Paper No. 10817 (2004)

4. Siewert, U., Fendrich, K., Doblhammer-Reiter, G., Scholz, R.D., Schuff-Werner, P., Hoffmann, W.: Health care consequences of demographic changes in Mecklenburg-West Pomerania: projected case numbers for age-related diseases up to the year 2020, based on the study of health in Pomerania (SHIP). Deutsches Ärzteblatt Int. **107**(18), 328 (2010)

5. Shaw, J.E., Sicree, R.A., Zimmet, P.Z.: Global estimates of the prevalence of diabetes for 2010 and 2030. Diabetes Res. Clin. Pract. **87**(1), 4–14 (2010)

6. Wild, S., Roglic, G., Green, A., Sicree, R., King, H.: Global prevalence of diabetes: estimates for the year 2000 and projections for 2030. Diabetes Care **27**(5), 1047–1053 (2004)

7. Roger, V.L., Go, A.S., Lloyd-Jones, D.M., Adams, R.J., Berry, J.D., Brown, T.M., American Heart Association Statistics Committee and Stroke Statistics Subcommittee: Heart disease and stroke statistics–2011 update: a report from the American Heart Association. Circulation **123**(4), e18–e209 (2004)

8. Poore, C.: Disability in Twentieth-Century German Culture. University of Michigan Press, Ann Arbor (2007)

9. World Health Organization (WHO): World Health Day 2012: ageing and health: toolkit for event organizers (2012). http://apps.who.int/iris/bitstream/10665/70840/1/WHO_DCO_WHD_2012.1_eng.pdf

10. Memon, M., Wagner, S.R., Pedersen, C.F., Beevi, F.H.A., Hansen, F.O.: Ambient assisted living healthcare frameworks, platforms, standards, and quality attributes. Sensors **14**(3), 4312–4341 (2014)

11. Frank, S., Labonnote, N.: Monitoring technologies for buildings equipped with ambient assisted living: current status and where next. In: SAI Intelligent Systems Conference (IntelliSys), pp. 431–438. IEEE (2015)

12. Cheng, J., Chen, X., Shen, M.: A framework for daily activity monitoring and fall detection based on surface electromyography and accelerometer signals. IEEE J. Biomed. Health Inform. **17**(1), 38–45 (2013)

13. Baig, M.M., Gholamhosseini, H.: Smart health monitoring systems: an overview of design and modeling. J. Med. Syst. **37**(2), 1–14 (2013)

14. Kleinberger, T., Becker, M., Ras, E., Holzinger, A., Müller, P.: Ambient intelligence in assisted living: enable elderly people to handle future interfaces. In: Stephanidis, C. (ed.) UAHCI 2007. LNCS, vol. 4555, pp. 103–112. Springer, Heidelberg (2007). https://doi.org/10.1007/978-3-540-73281-5_11

15. Rashidi, P., Mihailidis, A.: A survey on ambient-assisted living tools for older adults. IEEE J. Biomed. Health Inform. **17**(3), 579–590 (2013)

16. Wichert, R., Furfari, F., Kung, A., Tazari, M.R.: How to overcome the market entrance barrier and achieve the market breakthrough in AAL. In: Wichert, R., Eberhardt, B. (eds.) Ambient Assisted Living. ATSC, pp. 349–358. Springer, Heidelberg (2012). https://doi.org/10.1007/978-3-642-27491-6_25

17. Georgieff, P.: Ambient assisted living. Marktpotenziale IT-unterstützter Pflege für ein selbstbestimmtes Altern. [Market potential of IT-supported care for self-determined aging]. FAZIT Forschungsbericht **17**, 9–10 (2008)

18. Dohr, A., Modre-Opsrian, R., Drobics, M., Hayn, D., Schreier, G.: The Internet of Things for ambient assisted living. In: 2010 Seventh International Conference on Information Technology: New Generations (ITNG), pp. 804–809. IEEE (2010)

19. Stone, E.E., Skubic, M.: Fall detection in homes of older adults using the Microsoft Kinect. IEEE J. Biomed. Health Inform. **19**(1), 290–301 (2015)

20. Ni, B., Nguyen, C.D., Moulin, P.: RGBD-camera based get-up event detection for hospital fall prevention. In: International Conference on Acoustics, Speech and Signal Processing (ICASSP), pp. 1405–1408. IEEE (2012)
21. Costa, R., Novais, P., Costa, Â., Neves, J.: Memory support in ambient assisted living. In: Camarinha-Matos, L.M., Paraskakis, I., Afsarmanesh, H. (eds.) PRO-VE 2009. IAICT, vol. 307, pp. 745–752. Springer, Heidelberg (2009). https://doi.org/10.1007/978-3-642-04568-4_75
22. Hristova, A., Bernardos, A.M., Casar, J.R.: Context-aware services for ambient assisted living: a case-study. In: IEEE Applied Sciences on Biomedical and Communication Technologies, pp. 1–5 (2008)
23. Patel, S., Park, H., Bonato, P., Chan, L., Rodgers, M.: A review of wearable sensors and systems with application in rehabilitation. J. Neuroeng. Rehabil. 9(1), 21 (2012)
24. Essence Homepage: Smart Care - Care@ Home Product Suite (2018). http://www.essence-grp.com/smart-care/care-at-home-pers
25. Tunstall Homepage: Tunstall - Solutions for Healthcare Professionals (2018). https://uk.tunstall.com
26. Gövercin, M., Meyer, S., Schellenbach, M., Steinhagen-Thiessen, E., Weiss, B., Haesner, M.: SmartSenior@home: acceptance of an integrated ambient assisted living system. Results of a clinical field trial in 35 households. Inform. Health Soc. Care 41, 1–18 (2016)
27. Isern, D., Sánchez, D., Moreno, A.: Agents applied in health care: a review. Int. J. Med. Inform. 79(3), 145–166 (2010)
28. van Heek, J., Himmel, S., Ziefle, M.: Helpful but spooky? Acceptance of AAL-systems contrasting user groups with focus on disabilities and care needs'. In: Proceedings of the International Conference on ICT for Aging Well (ICT4AWE 2017), pp. 78–90. SCITEPRESS – Science and Technology Publications (2017)
29. Himmel, S., Ziefle, M.: Smart home medical technologies: users' requirements for conditional acceptance. I-Com 15(1), 39–50 (2016)
30. Beringer, R., Sixsmith, A., Campo, M., Brown, J., McCloskey, R.: The "acceptance" of ambient assisted living: developing an alternate methodology to this limited research lens. In: Abdulrazak, B., Giroux, S., Bouchard, B., Pigot, H., Mokhtari, M. (eds.) ICOST 2011. LNCS, vol. 6719, pp. 161–167. Springer, Heidelberg (2011). https://doi.org/10.1007/978-3-642-21535-3_21
31. Sun, H., De Florio, V., Gui, N., Blondia, C.: The missing ones: key ingredients towards effective ambient assisted living systems. J. Ambient Intell. Smart Environ. 2(2), 109–120 (2010)
32. Wilkowska, W., Ziefle, M.: Privacy and data security in e-health: requirements from users' perspective. Health Inform. J. 18(3), 191–201 (2012)
33. Wilkowska, W., Ziefle, M., Himmel, S.: Perceptions of personal privacy in smart home technologies: do user assessments vary depending on the research method? In: Tryfonas, T., Askoxylakis, I. (eds.) HAS 2015. LNCS, vol. 9190, pp. 592–603. Springer, Cham (2015). https://doi.org/10.1007/978-3-319-20376-8_53
34. van Heek, J., Himmel, S., Ziefle, M.: Privacy, data security, and the acceptance of AAL-systems – a user-specific perspective. In: Zhou, J., Salvendy, G. (eds.) ITAP 2017. LNCS, vol. 10297, pp. 38–56. Springer, Cham (2017). https://doi.org/10.1007/978-3-319-58530-7_4
35. Demiris, G., et al.: Older adults' attitudes towards and perceptions of "smart home" technologies: a pilot study. Med. Inform. Internet 29(2), 87–94 (2004)
36. Ziefle, M., Himmel, S., Wilkowska, W.: When your living space knows what you do: acceptance of medical home monitoring by different technologies. In: Holzinger, A., Simonic, K.-M. (eds.) USAB 2011. LNCS, vol. 7058, pp. 607–624. Springer, Heidelberg (2011). https://doi.org/10.1007/978-3-642-25364-5_43

37. Larizza, M.F., et al.: In-home monitoring of older adults with vision impairment: exploring patients', caregivers' and professionals' views. J. Am. Med. Inform. Assoc. **21**(1), 56–63 (2014)
38. López, S.A., Corno, F., Russis, L.D.: Supporting caregivers in assisted living facilities for persons with disabilities: a user study. Univ. Access Inf. Soc. **14**(1), 133–144 (2015)
39. Mortenson, W.B., Demers, L., Fuhrer, M.J., Jutai, J.W., Lenker, J., DeRuyter, F.: Effects of an assistive technology intervention on older adults with disabilities and their informal caregivers: an exploratory randomized controlled trial. Am. J. Phys. Med. Rehabil./Assoc. Acad. Physiatr. **92**(4), 297–306 (2013)
40. Ziefle, M., Jakobs, E.M.: New challenges in human computer interaction: strategic directions and interdisciplinary trends. In: 4th International Conference on Competitive Manufacturing Technologies, COMA, pp. 389–398 (2010)
41. Beier, G.: Kontrollüberzeugungen im Umgang mit Technik, [Control beliefs in dealing with technology]. Rep. Psychol. **9**, 684–693 (1999)
42. Xu, H., Dinev, T., Smith, H.J., Hart, P.: Examining the formation of individual's privacy concerns: toward an integrative view. In: ICIS 2008 Proceedings, p. 6 (2008)
43. Morton, A.: Measuring inherent privacy concern and desire for privacy-a pilot survey study of an instrument to measure dispositional privacy concern. In: International Conference on Social Computing (SocialCom), pp. 468–477. IEEE (2013)
44. McKnight, D.H., Choudhury, V., Kacmar, C.: Developing and validating trust measures for e-commerce: an integrative typology. Inf. Syst. Res. **13**(3), 334–359 (2002)
45. Van Heek, J., Ziefle, M., Himmel, S.: Caregivers' perspectives on ambient assisted living technologies in professional care contexts. In: Proceedings of the 4th International Conference on Information and Communication Technologies for Ageing Well and e-Health (ICT4AWE 2018), pp. 37–48 (2018)
46. Ziefle, M., Schaar, A.K.: Technical expertise and its influence on the acceptance of future medical technologies: what is influencing what to which extent? In: Leitner, G., Hitz, M., Holzinger, A. (eds.) USAB 2010. LNCS, vol. 6389, pp. 513–529. Springer, Heidelberg (2010). https://doi.org/10.1007/978-3-642-16607-5_40
47. Simonazzi, A.: Care regimes and national employment models. Camb. J. Econ. **33**(2), 211–232 (2008)

Playfully Assessing the Acceptance and Choice of Ambient Assisted Living Technologies by Older Adults

Eva-Maria Schomakers[✉], Julia Offermann-van Heek, and Martina Ziefle

Human-Computer Interaction Center, RWTH Aachen University,
Campus-Boulevard 57, Aachen, Germany
schomakers@comm.rwth-aachen.de
http://www.comm.rwth-aachen.de/

Abstract. Ambient Assisted Living (AAL) technologies have the potential to enable people in older age to stay home longer. Although the technological options increase steadily, the broad implementation of AAL technologies has failed so far. As reasons, a lack of availability of AAL end products on the market, missing trust in technologies, and a lack of acceptance are discussed. Previous empirical studies on the acceptance of AAL technologies mostly use impersonal online questionnaires referring to just one technology to evaluate without choice. To fully understand technology acceptance, it is of paramount importance that the participants can empathize with high-maintenance situations and that they are honest in their evaluations. Therefore, this paper aimed to develop a personal and playful assessment approach with regard to diverse AAL technologies using an interview study (n = 6) in the first step. In a second step, the developed playful approach was transferred to an online survey addressing older adults (n = 122). After presenting the results, their suitability, differences, and similarities are intensively discussed.

Keywords: Ambient Assisted Living · Technology acceptance · Assistive technology · Older adults · Playful assessment · Care scenarios

1 Introduction

Due to demographic change, the care sectors are under increasing pressure as more and more older people are in need of care [5,32]. Most older adults prefer to stay in their familiar and beloved home environment and wish to live independently as long as possible [34]. To support older people and people in need of care, more and more technological solutions are developed. Technologies assist in tasks of everyday life, support therapy and health management, and provide security in emergency situations. In the area of these so-called Ambient Assisted Living (AAL) technologies, there have been many developments in the last decades [21] and multiple holistic systems as well as single-case solutions are

© Springer Nature Switzerland AG 2019
P. D. Bamidis et al. (Eds.): ICT4AWE 2018, CCIS 982, pp. 26–44, 2019.
https://doi.org/10.1007/978-3-030-15736-4_2

in the testing stage and partly also available on the market [6, 26]. Resounding success and frequent usage of these innovative AAL technologies in home environments have failed to appear so far [33]. Technology acceptance by the users represent one of the greatest barriers for market success [22].

Previous research on the acceptance of AAL technologies applied mostly interviews or online questionnaires. The use of scenarios or system prototypes is common, but mostly those artificial situations are impersonal and do not get people, who are not (yet) in need of care, to empathize with high-maintenance situations, and to evaluate systems and technologies accordingly in regard to their own lives.

In this paper, we report and compare two innovative methodological approaches. First, in game-based interviews, we playfully assessed the wishes, perceived barriers, and perceived benefits of older adults regarding AAL technologies (see also [27]). This approach was then transferred to an online questionnaire with open questions, thus reaching a wider sample of older adults and providing an anonymous environment for them to express their wishes, needs, and concerns. In this paper, the results of the game-based online questionnaire are reported.

2   AAL Technologies and Acceptance

We start by summarizing the state of the art concerning AAL technologies, before presenting the theoretical background of technology acceptance research focusing on AAL technologies. Further, the approach of the current studies and our research aims are outlined.

2.1   Ambient Assisted Living

Since the 1980s, Information and Communication Technologies (ICT) have been discussed to be used in everyday life [28]. By using and integrating ICT (e.g., cameras or movement sensors) within home environments, assistance and monitoring were made possible. The term Ambient Assisted Living (AAL) refers to the use of technologies to assist older people in aging-in-place, supporting living independently, staying active, remaining socially connected and mobile [4]. AAL technologies come as applications, devices as well as holistic AAL systems covering a wide range of different use cases and technologies. Some of these systems are currently available for an integration in private home environments (e.g., [6, 13]) or are developed and improved in current research activities (e.g., [14, 29]).

AAL technologies cover different aspects of life: One prominent type of technology for enhancing safety are personal alarm and monitoring systems, especially for the case of falls of older adults [7, 9]. Supporting social life and communication for staying connected with friends, family, and caregivers is another aim of AAL technologies. Further, the chores of daily living can be facilitated with automated technologies, such as home automation or memory aids (e.g., [16]). And these, are only a few exemplary use cases.

Many AAL technologies focus on elderly people and their needs in general, but also more and more technologies are developed to assist people with special needs. For example, much research is conducted to support people with dementia in private home but also in professional care contexts [12].

The number of available AAL systems and research projects is high and increases steadily. Although these technologies have the potential to facilitate everyday life of older adults, they are not yet widely used. Technology acceptance by older adults - the potential users - represents one of the decisive barriers against a widespread adoption of AAL technologies [22].

2.2   Technology Acceptance

Most studies on technology acceptance are based on the Technology Acceptance Model (TAM) [10] and the Unified Theory of Acceptance and Use of Technology (UTAUT) [31]. In these models, the intention to adopt a technology is mainly explained by the Perceived Usefulness and the Perceived Ease of Use. The UTAUT model also includes the influences of facilitating conditions, social influence, and moderating factors (Age, Gender, Experience, and Voluntariness of Use). These models might explain technology adoption sufficiently in a variety of contexts but are mostly concentrated on job-related applications and consumer electronics.

AAL technologies aim at the diverse and special group of older adults, provide a diversity of technical system (from stand-alone devices, smartphone applications, to ubiquitous systems), and are applied in very intimate, medical, and therapeutic contexts within the beloved home environment. Correspondingly, additional motives and barriers need to be taken into account (e.g., [8,18,24]). Older adults mostly acknowledge the usefulness and necessity of technology support in several areas. Benefits include e.g., the social connectedness, health and safety, support with daily activities, or education [19]. Also the release of burden of family and caregivers plays an important role. Still, many concerns are prevalent. The most relevant are concerns regarding privacy intrusion, a low usability of the system, and high purchase and maintenance costs as well as the lack of perceived benefits [18,24]. Potential users weigh up the benefits and barriers. These trade-offs are decisive for the decision to use an AAL system within an individual (care) situation [15].

2.3   Assessment of Technology Acceptance

Most research on the acceptance of AAL technologies by older adults uses qualitative methodologies like interviews and focus groups [24]. Qualitative studies are suited to deeply understand the participants motives and attitudes, and thus, are adequate for identifying motives and barriers. In most qualitative studies, scenarios and presentations are used to describe the technology, or the participants can interact with (a prototype of) the systems. Recently, some approaches have been made to include older adults into the design process via participatory design approaches (e.g., [14,23]). A multitude of motives, barriers, and wishes of older adults has been identified by qualitative research in the past [24]; however, qualitative studies are limited to small sample sizes. Additionally, face-to-face interviews may result in biased responses, e.g., responses strongly influenced by social desirability as an emotional bond between interviewer and interviewee is formed.

In quantitative studies, the relative extent of the influence of barriers and benefits and the influence of user diversity factors, e.g., age, health status, or gender, can be assessed with a larger sample. Comparability between contexts, scenarios, as well as technologies can be achieved. The results may be generalized and are often seen as more objective. Most quantitative approaches nowadays use online surveys with scenarios and technology descriptions. Mostly, close-ended questions and ratings are used. Correspondingly, insights are restricted to a quantification of the given questions, comprehension problems can possibly occur, and the situation may be artificial and impersonal. Especially in such an intimate topic as assistive technologies, empathy with the described situations and a deeper understanding of the motives and trade-offs are very important. Thus, close-ended questionnaires can be limiting.

That the methodological approaches influence the results and the evaluation of benefits and barriers of novel technologies was shown by Wilkowska and colleagues [35]. They conducted a comparison of methodological approaches to measure privacy concerns in an assistive environment and illustrated that the relative importance of privacy concerns for the participants varied across the applied research methods. In a hands-on experiment, the importance of privacy aspects was significantly lower compared to questionnaire studies and focus groups. Apparently, the mere vision to use such a system (as applied in questionnaires and focus groups) led to an overestimation of potential privacy issues, while interacting with the system helps people to build trust, without primarily concentrating on potential privacy intrusion.

2.4 Our Approach

In this publication, we report the results of two game-based research approaches to assess the acceptance of assistive technologies. A procedure related to a board game was developed in which the participants are presented with several scenarios and use cases for assistive technologies and are asked to choose between different technologies.

Nowadays, more and more assistive technologies are on the market and older adults need not only decide whether to use a technology, but also which technology to use. The process of choosing between different technology options can reveal additional insights into older adults' wishes and needs as well as their evaluation criteria. Still, the decision whether to use technology at all in a given scenario is included into our method. Additional details may emerge in comparison between the technologies. Moreover, the participants are not biased by the thought that one does not want to speak ill about the system an interviewer or questionnaire is presenting as there are several options.

We aimed to create an approach that combines the advantages of both qualitative and quantitative methods and that, at the same time, brings participants into a playful but realistic situation in which they can empathize with the given scenarios and freely share their opinions. In both, the offline and the online approach, scenarios and technologies are visualized to make them more realistic. The task to choose between technologies is close to the purchase decision situation in real life. This approach has been tested offline in personal interviews with 6 older adults (cf. [27]) and was then transferred to an online survey approach using still the same game based elements and open-ended questions. In this paper, the results of the online questionnaire approach are reported and compared to the interview results.

3   Method

In this section, the online version of our game-based method is explained in more detail. In summer 2017, six personal interviews with older adults functioned as a prestudy for this new game-based approach. These qualitative results and a detailed description of the method can be found in [27]. As this prestudy proved very useful and worth a follow up, the elements of the interview were transferred to an online questionnaire instrument with the aim to maintain the playful character and qualitative assessment of barriers and benefits.

3.1   The Game

Central to both, the interviews and the online questionnaire, is a game of choosing technology options. The participants are presented with five to six different technology options for each use case—from which they can choose their most preferred technology as well the one that they reject the most. Reasoning and motives for the respective decisions are then asked with an open-ended question to receive in-depth answers. In the 'offline' prestudy, the participants were asked to tell the interviewer their reasoning. In the online questionnaire, they were invited to describe their motives in a text field explaining their choice.

This choice task is repeated several times. At the beginning, the participants are asked to put themselves into a scenario of living alone in older age. All use cases are then gone through one time. Afterwards, the scenario changes to one with higher needs for support and the participants are asked to rethink the choices in each use case and to state whether there are differences in their choice and reasoning.

In the 'offline' prestudy, the participants were presented with 6 different use cases of assistive technology. Of these, each two were similar and used the same technology options to reduce the complexity and memory load for the participants. For the online study, two central use cases were selected that showed to be quite different in their assessment in the prestudy. The scenarios, use cases, and technology options of the online study are described in detail in the following.

3.2   The Scenarios

The participants were asked to put themselves into the following two scenarios. Always, the first scenario of "moderate need for support" was presented first, as the scenario "higher need for support" is based on the first one.

Scenario "moderate need for support":

Please imagine yourself in the following scenario: You are 71 years old, living alone in your familiar home environment. You are in retirement for a few years now and enjoy your retired life. Recently, you realize more and more that your daily chores are getting harder to cope with, as you are troubled with small health problems. Still, you can carry out most tasks on your own, but it happens more frequently that you feel somewhat overtaxed. Your family is unable to support you as much as they would like to, as they are living far away. Thus, you are mostly on your own in your daily life.

Scenario "higher need for support":

Please imagine that 10 years have passed: You are now older than 80 years and still live alone in your home. Unfortunately, a severe chronic illness has taken hold of you in the last years, which causes you to feel unsteady and wobbly on your legs. Recently, you have fallen several times and, afterwards, you have had troubles getting up again. Luckily, you have not been seriously hurt until now. Additionally, problems with disorientation and forgetfulness are steadily increasing. For your support, a nursing service attends you every morning for half an hour. They assist you with getting up, getting dressed, and your physical hygiene, but leave you alone afterwards until the next day. For the rest of your day, you are on your own.

The scenarios were chosen to appeal to most older adults as no specific disease is addressed but a general, age-related frailness and forgetfulness. Further, the scenarios were visualized with a drawing of the face of an older adult with the gender matching that of the interviewee to make it more appealing and help the participants to empathize with the text.

3.3   The Use Cases and Technology Options

Two opposing use cases were chosen. The first one, fall detection, represents an application area of assistive technology, that is used in rare and sudden emergency cases that can have severe consequences, whereas medical reminders support everyday tasks in a medical, therapeutic context. For the introduction to the use cases, a short text explained why it is important in older age to be supported with these tasks and gave illustrative examples. The technology options were provided with a short description of how they can be applied within the use case and were additionally visualized with neutral clip-art images for better understanding and memorizing (cf. Fig. 1).

Fall Detection: For the fall detection use case, the example of sudden falls is given, in which the older adult does not get up on its own anymore and needs to

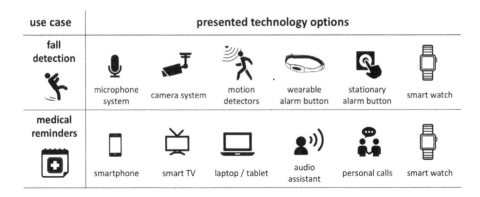

Fig. 1. Presented technologies options in both use cases, fall detection and medical reminders.

raise an alarm. The following technology options were presented to the participants: stationary alarm buttons, wearable alarm buttons, smart watches, microphone systems, camera systems, and motion detectors.

Medical Reminders: Examples for medical reminders were reminders to take medication, to measure vital parameters like blood pressure or weight, as well as to go to medical appointments, to make new appointments, and get new prescriptions when needed. The participants could chose between the following technology options: smartphone, smart TV, laptop/tablet, audio assistant, personal calls, and smart watch.

3.4   Structure of the Questionnaire

The online questionnaire consisted of three parts. At first, demographic data (age, gender, educational level) were enquired. Before the game started, also attitudes towards aging, technology, and privacy were assessed. The participants evaluated their *attitude towards aging* [3], their *technical self-efficacy* (abridged scale by [1]), as well as their *disposition to value privacy* [36]. All items were assessed on a 6-point Likert scale ranging from "I do not agree at all" (1) to "I fully agree" (6). After assessing these individual characteristics, the participants were introduced to the game with the first scenario and use case. The order of the use cases was randomized. At the end, the participants shortly evaluated how well they could empathize with the scenarios on a one-item scale ranging from "very easy to empathize with" to "very abstract".

3.5   The Analysis

The written comments were analyzed within the framework of a content analysis. The coding scheme of the prestudy was reapplied for the analysis of the online study, thus, using a directed approach [17]. Still, new categories were added when new topics emerged in the comments. The categories consist of the perceived barriers and benefits of the presented technologies, as well as motives and conditions the participants mentioned to chose technologies as preferred or most rejected ones. They are structured as thematic areas. For example, missing ease of use as a barrier, good ease of use as a benefit, as well as good ease of use as a conditional requirement were all coded into the category "ease of use". This proved useful because the participants did not only use absolute evaluations (e.g., this violates my privacy) but in the comparison of technologies also relative evaluations have been made (e.g., it is still privacy-invasive, but better than the other technology).

Two coders went over the material several times. As the study was carried out in German, the native language of the participants, quotes selected for publication are translated to English.

4   The Sample

$N = 122$ adults older than 50 years completed the online questionnaire. They were recruited via the authors' social network and through snow ball recruiting. The participants' mean age was 60.4 years, with 63% women, and 37% men. 73% of participants reported to hold a university degree showing a generally high education level. Still, other educational levels were also present in the study. The participants were slightly confident regarding their abilities to interact with technology (technical self-efficacy: $M = 4.14$, $SD = 1.12$) and reported to be rather neutral regarding their need for privacy (privacy disposition: $M = 3.79$, $SD = .94$). The participants' attitude towards aging was positive on average ($M = 4.36$, $SD = 0.57$).

5   Results

The results part is structured as follows: first the barriers and benefits of fall detection technologies are presented. Then, medical reminders are examined. For each use case, the two scenarios are contrasted. A comparison between the offline prestudy and these online results follows.

In summary, 75% of respondents gave reasonable answers to our questions (362 comments in total) which resulted in 528 codings. Thus, the participants showed a high motivation in answering our questions. A counting of the codings per category is illustrated in Fig. 2 for both use cases and scenarios.

5.1   Barriers and Benefits to Use Fall Detection Technologies

Scenario "Moderate need for support": The main goal and thus a very important aspect was the **effectiveness** of the technology in detecting falls and increasing security. Also, two thirds of the participants addressed **privacy implications** as an essential barrier for fall detection technology, especially camera systems.

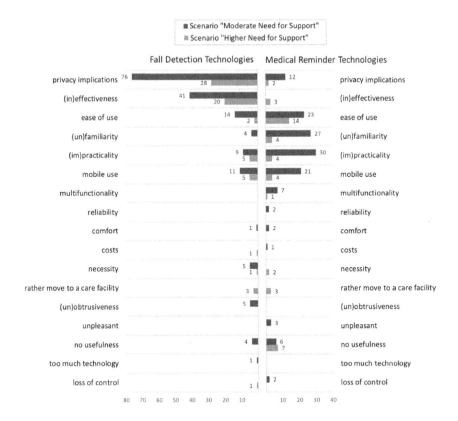

Fig. 2. Number of comments relating to the themes in comparison between both use cases and scenarios (total number of comments = 362, total number of codings = 528).

Most participants stated that they would feel surveilled by the technology, which is uncomfortable to them. Two participants were also concerned regarding data protection. The effectiveness of a technology was weighed up against the privacy implications. The participants preferred the technology that they deemed as most effective and which they can still tolerate in its privacy violations. This privacy-utility trade-off was prevalent in many comments.

> *"I want maximum support in emergency situations with as little reduction of privacy/technical surveillance as possible"*
> *"I think an emergency button provides fast help in emergencies without me feeling surveilled. The other options provide too much surveillance, violate my privacy too much."*
> *"Basic security by simple technology: emergency button. The individual costs (challenge of interacting with the technology, feeling of surveillance) of a permanent camera monitoring is too high for the presented scenario."*

Related to the effectiveness of a technology, the possibility of a **mobile use** also outside of the home was mentioned as important benefits in 11 comments.

> *"Smart watch: would probably be also helpful when I fall in the garden."*
> *"With the smart watch I feel more free and independent, because I can also raise an alarm in case of an emergency outside of my apartment."*

Further, a specific technology was chosen because it was generally the most **practical** in one's personal daily life and thus, practicality was mentioned as an important condition by 9 participants:

> *"Smart watch: does not bother me in my daily duties and is always on my arm"*

The topic **ease of use** was addressed by 14 participants. Some chose a technology that they thought would be most easy to use, others imposed ease of use as a condition:

> *"Simple interaction [...] speaks in favour for the smart watch."*
> *"Especially for emergencies, the smart watch convinces me. For decades, I have been wearing a watch. If it can detect falls and provides functions to raise an alarm, that would be very nice, provided that it is easy to use."*

Closely related to the ease of use, the **familiarity** with the technology was mentioned by 4 participants:

> *"The watch is a medium that I am familiar with."*
> *"I am already wearing a smart watch, so no adjustments/conversion would be necessary."*

Also important to the participants in the online questionnaire was **autonomy** in raising an alarm, thus rejecting automatic detection.

> *"The emergency button can be wilfully activated (only when needed)."*
> *"I think the emergency button is most appropriate, as one can decide one-self whether help is needed."*

The only comment regarding **comfort** as benefit of technology represented a very general praise to technology.

> *"Technologies provide valuable support and freedom, and comfort."*

As new topic, the **unobtrusiveness** of the smart watch emerged and was mentioned as a potential benefit by five participants. Under the theme **no usefulness**, comments were coded that denied the presented technologies any usefulness. Three participants thought that there are better alternatives than the presented technologies, e.g., by using a phone. One participant stated: *"Everybody has to die sometime.* Arguments of this kind were also identified during the prestudy. Similarly, four participants shared the opinion that in the scenario "moderate need for support" technological support was **not yet necessary**, e.g.: *"Honestly, I can't see that I already need technological support in this scenario."*

Scenario "Higher Need for Support". 36 participants did not see changes in their reasoning for the second scenario that portrays oneself being older, frail, and in need for care. For others, the above described privacy calculus of weighing the benefits with the **privacy implications** did now result in the acceptance of more privacy invasive technologies:

> *"The security and the protection [the technology offers] would probably be increasingly more relevant than the protection of my privacy"*
> *"The protection of my privacy has become less important, more important however is fast medical care and security."*
> *"The older I grow the more I am dependent on technology to detect emergencies, even if my privacy is thereby violated."*

Ease of use, **mobile use**, and **practicality** issues were mentioned again by some participants. One participant states that it would also be *"a matter of money"*. Also, again **autonomy** in raising the alarm was mentioned:

> *"I can always wear the emergency button around the wrist and get help when I need it. I am in control of the process, I decide whether and when I press the button."*

Only three participants stated that they would not want to live at home any more in case of this scenario and would **rather move into a care facility** or a retirement community.

> *"I think that I would move into a retirement community or similar in this scenario of heavy limitations."*

5.2   Barriers and Benefits to Use Medical Reminders

Scenario of "Moderate Need for Support". For the decision which technology to use for medical reminders, two important thematic areas emerged: the ease of use, that is related to the familiarity with the technology, and practicality issues that include mobile use as well as multifunctionality of the technology.

Several aspects for the **ease of use** of the presented technologies are addressed by the participants. The **familiarity** with a technology was seen as important in order to be able to interact with it especially in older age when the learning of new technologies becomes harder. But also the auditory, visual, and motor skills decrease in older age, so that buttons and displays should not be too small and audio signals may be overheard.

> *"The support of the presented use case, e.g., by a smartphone, is only then reasonable when the interaction with such devices has been learned in younger age. [...] If one gets more forgetful in older age, one cannot acquire the use of apps as easy as in younger age. [...] But the technology and interaction with technology develops all the time and I figure that, from a certain age on, I won't be able to cope with these developments. That's why the presented solutions will only work when they are very easy*

to use. [...] Moreover, you have to consider that older people often have poor hearing and eyesight. The interaction with a smart watch is therefore not possible at all because of the small screen. The screen is often to small even on smartphones."

"The smartphone is the most familiar for me and is also already important in my daily life. The audio assistant is unknown to me and may be also harder to interact with."

Further important aspects referred to habits and how a technology could be integrated into everyday life, leading to **practicality** issues. For reminders, it was seen as important to be reminded wherever one is (**mobile use**) and the device should therefore be always close and always switched on. For some participants it was also important to use a device they already use for other functions, so that no additional device is needed (**multifunctionality**).

"With starting forgetfulness, the smart phone could be mislaid. Computer and TV are not present in every room and may not be heard. A smart watch can be programmed by me or an assisting person, it is worn at the body, but should be waterproof and not removable."

"The smart watch is worn at the wrist, it is quick, just once a morning you have to think about putting it on, it does not bother me in my daily life. The smart TV is too laborious and is only reasonable when I visit this room now and then."

Additionally, **privacy implications** were addressed by the participants. As in the case of emergency technologies, a feeling of surveillance was mentioned. But more prevalent than in the other use case concerns regarding data protection were expressed:

"I think that regarding all these questions it is decisive in which political system we will live at that time. With good data protection and security and a governmental atmosphere that is friendly to the ill and old, I can image that the presented technology are of great use."

"The audio assistant reminds me of 'Big Brother"'.

Two participants addressed technology being **comfortable** as another decision criteria. Only one participant addressed the **costs** of the devices. Two participants found the presented technology solutions as "too much control and dependence on technology." Moreover, technology should be **reliable**. The voice of an audioassistant was thought to be **unpleasant**.

Six participants saw **no use** in the technology in this use case and scenario. They stated, that they still want to use their brain and that this is also important in older age.

"I am 88 years old [...] I want to use my mind and it still works."

"In the presented scenario, I cannot see an important factor to use technology. In this situation, I consider it rather useful to care for oneself without technologies."

Scenario "Higher Need for Support": Again, the change of the scenario did not change the decision criteria for one third of the participants (38 statements). Within the other comments, a shift can be observed that practicality was less often mentioned (4 comments), but ease of use relatively more often (14 comments). Comments regarding the **ease of use** stressed that it is the most decisive condition as in a scenario of forgetfulness and frailty some technologies cannot be used anymore at all. For some participants this led to the assessment that all these technologies are of no use due to the inability to interact with them.

> *"The audio assistant is very unreliable when you cannot hear well anymore."*
> *"Because in older age I would probably be not able to use a smart phone (forgetting where it is, too small display). [...] The smart watch would be surely too small (decreased eyesight)."*
> *"But when I am forgetful and more, I won't be able to interact with any technology so that all technology is for nothing."*

Familiarity with the technology was mentioned again as one factor that leads to the ability to interact with a technology, but was also not as often mentioned as in the first scenario.

The comments regarding **practicality** were also related to the handling of the technology. They discussed, e.g., too small screens, not loud enough audio signals, and also the ability to put on a watch, e.g.: *"smart watch: who will put it on? Display and interaction elements too small."* Also, only four participants still addressed a **mobile use** as criteria for technology choice. A **multifunctional** technology was wished for by one participant.

Privacy implications, in particular data protection concerns, were only mentioned by two participants as a barrier. Other participants stated that in this scenario of increased necessity the most important criteria was for the technology to work effectively and that *"need for security and wish for autonomy let all other criteria recede into the background."*

Again, the three same participants (similar to the use case of fall detection) stated that they would **rather move to a care facility** in this scenario than to be home alone.

5.3   Comparison to the Results of the Prestudy

Most of the thematic areas have already been addressed by the participants in the prestudy. New to the analysis were the aspects *reliability, (un)obtrusiveness* as well as *unpleasant* and *too much technology*. These areas were each addressed by not more than four participants. Three participants choosing to go to a nursing home in the second scenario than to live alone at home represented also a new aspect in comparison to the prestudy.

In comparison between the use cases, privacy implications and effectiveness were most often mentioned for fall detection technologies, whereas ease of use and practicality issues are more often addressed regarding medical reminder technologies. Similar countings were already observed in the prestudy.

Comparing the two scenarios, we also saw similar shifts in the prestudy and this study. Overall, the participants mentioned fewer aspects in the scenario of "higher need for support" than in the first one. This effect may have several causes. On the one hand, the order of the scenarios was not randomized so that the participants could be weary. Also maybe, they did not want to repeat themselves too much and just mentioned the most decisive aspects again. On the other hand, it can also be hypothesized that in a scenario of greater necessity to get support, some aspects are not important anymore, e.g., technology being comfortable and pleasant to use. This hypothesis is supported by the results of the prestudy in which participants addressed this directly.

A clear difference between the scenarios can be seen in the trade-off between privacy implications and the benefits of the technology in the use case of fall detection technologies. Privacy implications were also often mentioned in the second scenario, but they were mostly considered as outweighed by the security that the technology offers. Regarding medical reminders, the aspect of ease of use became more urgent for the scenario of "higher need for support". It was not anymore just annoying if a technology is hard to interact with, but older adults in this situation might not be able to use some technologies at all when no special effort is put into ergonomics and usability.

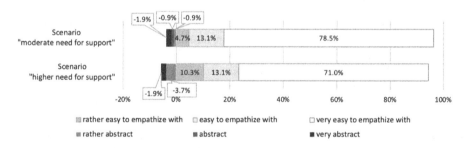

Fig. 3. Evaluation of the two scenarios: percentage of respondents attributing the levels from "very easy to empathize with" to "very abstract" with each scenario (N = 122).

5.4 Evaluation of the Scenarios

As a control of the method, we assessed how well the participants could empathize with the scenarios. For the first scenario, "moderate need for support", 78.5% of the participants stated that they found it very easy to acquaint themselves with. Only 2.8% of participants found the scenario rather abstract or abstract. The second scenario of "higher need for support" was slightly harder to acquaint with. 71% of the participants found it very easy to empathize with, whereas 4.6% judged it as (rather) abstract (cf. Fig. 3). All in all, this evaluation shows that the scenarios were easy to empathize with for the great majority of the participants.

6 Discussion and Conclusion

This paper presented a playful approach to the assessment of AAL acceptance criteria. A game-based interview approach [27] was transferred to an online questionnaire environment, using a qualitative approach with open-ended questions. The research aim was to assess motives and barriers of older adults (>50 years old) when choosing between different AAL technologies. Two use cases, namely, fall detection and medical reminders, with each six technology options, as well as two scenarios, one of "moderate need for support" and one of "higher need for support", were compared. The participants chose their most preferred and their most rejected technology option for each use case and scenario and commented on why they preferred/rejected this technology. Benefits, barriers, and conditions were identified in a content analysis. The online questionnaire was realized as appealing as possible and all technology options, as well as the scenario and use case descriptions were visualized.

There have been many studies identifying acceptance criteria of AAL technologies (e.g., [24]). In this study, no additional motives and barriers could be identified. However, the playful approach and to let participants choose between technology alternatives identified a shift of relevance of known barriers and benefits and a new angle to them.

6.1 Context- and Care-Specific AAL Acceptance

In the use case of fall detection, the trade-off between the effectiveness of the technology in detecting falls and raising an alarm is weighed up with privacy implications (that are prevalent especially with microphone and camera monitoring technologies). This *privacy calculus* results in privacy concerns hindering the use of the more privacy-invasive technologies within the first scenario. But when the necessity changes with the introduction of the second scenario, the participants still see the privacy implications, but these are overridden by the need for security and technology support. This cost-benefit calculation has been labeled privacy calculus and has been extensively studied in other contexts (e.g., [11,20]). Regarding the acceptance of AAL technologies, the privacy calculus has already been addressed [15], but needs to be examined further. For example, the question at what point the necessity of support and the benefits of the technology overrides privacy implications is very essential. Also, a better insight into which aspects of the technology raises privacy concerns seems relevant.

The decision criteria for medical reminders differ more between the two scenarios than in the case of fall detection technologies. For the first scenario, practicality and also ease of use are most important for medical reminders as it has also been found in previous empirical research [24]. Technologies need to be integrated into the users' everyday life and should not bother. Also, a mobile use is important. Additionally, technology should be easy to use. Most older adults prefer technology that they are already familiar with. Thus, in this scenario AAL systems and products need to focus on the practicability and match for the users' everyday life. Nowadays, many ICT devices already exist in older people's households. If possible, applications should work on the already existing devices which the users know how to interact with.

In the second scenario, a shift can be observed that ease of use is the main condition for acceptance and practicality issues decrease in importance. The participants argue that some technology options, e.g., the smart watch, are not usable in the described scenario. In older age, motor, audio, and visual skills decrease so that the interaction with technology becomes harder. Additionally, it is more difficult for older adults to learn to interact with new devices. Thus, technology in this scenario needs to be intuitively usable and should be developed so that older adults can easily interact with them [25]. No new interaction method but those that the technology generation is familiar with should be used.

At the same time, the comparison between technologies leads to new benefits in a way that being less privacy-invasive or more comfortable than other alternatives become perceived benefits and barriers. Therefore, the categories cannot be divided into barriers and benefits per se, but are rather thematic areas that can be a barrier or a benefits depending on the comparison.

Still, the most important aspect is that the technology can fulfill its function, e.g., reliably detect falls and remind of medical tasks as it is modeled within the conventional technology acceptance models (e.g., [10,31]). In most comments, this can be read between the lines and can also be seen in the categories. For example, the problem with practicality and usability issues is that if they occur the technology cannot be fully effective. However, if the users consider effectiveness as given other barriers and benefits become more foreground.

One insightful new aspect has been identified in this study: With the comparison of the two scenarios, the participants stressed the influence of the necessity to the choice of technology. Still, with the introduction of the second scenario, three participants stated that they would rather move into a care facility. Although a minority of other participants did not see the support by technology as an option, only 2.5% saw an alternative in being institutionalized. This illustrates again the wish for independent living at home, and correspondingly, how important the development of ambient assisting technology is.

6.2 Limitations

This new methodological approach proved useful for the evaluation of barriers and benefits of AAL technology and added a new perspective compared to previous research approaches. With the comparison between different technology options - a situation that is rather realistic at times in which more and more AAL technology are available - the relative relevance of the benefits and barriers as well as the trade-offs between them become more obvious. The playful approach with personal scenarios and visualization proved to be appealing, as the evaluation of the scenarios shows. Also, the high response rate and the very thought-out comments show that the participants put effort into answering the questions. Compared to the prestudy in which the same game was incorporated into interviews, no arguments were missing and even additional aspects were mentioned. Thus, this online approach with open-ended questions did not limit the range of aspects that the participants addressed. Rather, the participants seemed to be very honest as the answers were anonymous.

With our approach, we succeeded in combining the advantages of deep insights of qualitative studies with the opportunities of online questionnaires to reach a larger and more heterogeneous sample of older adults. Still, no quantitative approach was used and the countings of codings can only be descriptively and cautiously used to assess the relevance of the aspects [2]. To compare scenarios, use cases, and the relevance of the barriers and benefits, a quantitative method is still needed. With the use of choice-based conjoint experiments, also the trade-offs between privacy implications and perceived benefits of AAL technologies could be analyzed further.

Finally, there are also some limitations with regard to the sample of the present study. The study's sample size was sufficient in particular as it aimed for opinions, wishes, and requirements expressed by older adults. However, the study should be replicated in more representative samples, especially with regard to the participants' educational level: as the participants of the current study were highly educated, future studies should aim for a more balanced sample including higher proportions of people with a lower level of education. Further, the online study reached - of course - mostly technically-affine participants. For future studies, pencil-and-paper questionnaires should additionally be used in order to reach also participants who are not able or willing to fill out online questionnaires. Then, it will also be possible to investigate fringe groups (e.g., technically affine vs. not technically affine participants - being not online). As a last sample-related aspect, it has to be mentioned that the present study was conducted in Germany and represents a perspective of one single and specific country. In particular with regard to the privacy calculus, previous research has already shown country and culture differences in the evaluation of privacy [30]. Therefore, future studies should aim for a comparison of personal evaluations of AAL technologies focusing especially on the perception of the trade-off between potential benefits and barriers depending on different countries, cultures, backgrounds, and structures (e.g., policy, health care).

Acknowledgements. We thank all participants for their openness in sharing their opinions. Furthermore, the authors want to thank Nils Plettenberg and Susanne Gohr for their valuable research support. This work was funded by the German Federal Ministry of Education and Research, under the project Whistle (16SV7530) and the project MyneData (KIS1DSD045).

References

1. Beier, G.: Kontrollüberzeugungen im Umgang mit Technik [technical self-efficacy]. Rep. Psychol. **9**, 684–693 (1999)
2. Berelson, B.: Content Analysis in Communication Research. Free Press, New York (1952)

3. Biermann, H., Himmel, S., Offermann-van Heek, J., Ziefle, M.: User-specific concepts of aging – a qualitative approach on AAL-acceptance regarding ultrasonic whistles. In: Zhou, J., Salvendy, G. (eds.) ITAP 2018. LNCS, vol. 10927, pp. 231–249. Springer, Cham (2018). https://doi.org/10.1007/978-3-319-92037-5_18

4. Blackman, S., et al.: Ambient assisted living technologies for aging well: a scoping review. J. Intell. Syst. **25**(1), 55–69 (2016)

5. Bloom, D.E., Canning, D.: Global demographic change: dimensions and economic significance. Technical report, National Bureau of Economic Research (2004)

6. Casenio: Homepage: Casenio - Intelligente Hilfe- & Komfortsysteme [intelligent support and comfort systems] (2016). www.casenio.de

7. Chaudhuri, S., Thompson, H., Demiris, G.: Fall detection devices and their use with older adults: a systematic review. J. Geriatr. Phys. Tehr. **37**(4), 178–196 (2014)

8. Chen, K., Chan, A.H.S.: Review a review of technology acceptance by older adults. Gerontechnology **10**(1), 1–12 (2011)

9. Cheng, J., Chen, X., Shen, M.: A framework for daily activity monitoring and fall detection based on surface electromyography and accelerometer signals. IEEE J. Biomed. Health Inf. **17**(1), 38–45 (2013)

10. Davis, F.D.: Perceived usefulness, perceived ease of use, and user acceptance of information technology. MIS Q. **13**(3), 319–340 (1989)

11. Dinev, T., Hart, P.: An extended privacy calculus model for E-commerce transactions. Inf. Syst. Res. **17**(1), 61–80 (2006)

12. D'Onofrio, G., et al.: Information and communication technologies for the activities of daily living in older patients with dementia: a systematic review. J. Alzheimer's Dis. **57**(3), 927–935 (2017)

13. Essence Homepage: Smart care - care@home product suite (2016). http://www.essence-grp.com/smart-care/care-at-home-pers

14. Gövercin, M., Meyer, S., Schellenbach, M., Steinhagen-Thiessen, E., Weiss, B., Haesner, M.: SmartSenior@home: acceptance of an integrated ambient assisted living system results of a clinical field trial in 35 households. Inf. Health Soc. Care **41**, 1–18 (2016)

15. van Heek, J., Himmel, S., Ziefle, M.: Privacy, data security, and the acceptance of AAL-systems – a user-specific perspective. In: Zhou, J., Salvendy, G. (eds.) ITAP 2017. LNCS, vol. 10297, pp. 38–56. Springer, Cham (2017). https://doi.org/10.1007/978-3-319-58530-7_4

16. Hristova, A., Bernardos, A.M., Casar, J.R.: Context-aware services for ambient assisted living: a case-study. In: 2008 First International Symposium on Applied Sciences on Biomedical and Communication Technologies, ISABEL 2008, pp. 1–5. IEEE (2008)

17. Hsieh, H.F., Shannan, S.E.: Three approaches to qualitative content analysis. Qual. Health Res. **15**(9), 1277–1288 (2005)

18. Jaschinski, C., Allouch, S.B.: An extended view on benefits and barriers of ambient assisted living solutions. Int. J. Adv. Life Sci. **7**(1–2), 40–53 (2015)

19. Jaschinski, C., Ben Allouch, S.: Why should I use this? Identifying incentives for using AAL technologies. In: De Ruyter, B., Kameas, A., Chatzimisios, P., Mavrommati, I. (eds.) AmI 2015. LNCS, vol. 9425, pp. 155–170. Springer, Cham (2015). https://doi.org/10.1007/978-3-319-26005-1_11

20. Laufer, R.S., Wolfe, M.: Privacy as a concept and a social issue: a multidimensional developmental theory. J. Soc. Issues **33**(3), 22–42 (1977)

21. Memon, M., Wagner, S.R., Pedersen, C.F., Beevi, F.H.A., Hansen, F.O.: Ambient assisted living healthcare frameworks, platforms, standards, and quality attributes. Sensors **14**(3), 4312–4341 (2014)
22. Mollenkopf, H.: Enhancing Mobility in Later Life: Personal Coping, Environmental Resources and Technical Support; the Out-of-Home Mobility of Older Adults in Urban and Rural Regions of Five European Countries, vol. 17. IOS Press, Amsterdam (2005)
23. Muñoz, D., Gutierrez, F.J., Ochoa, S.F.: Introducing ambient assisted living technology at the home of the elderly: challenges and lessons learned. In: Cleland, I., Guerrero, L., Bravo, J. (eds.) IWAAL 2015. LNCS, vol. 9455, pp. 125–136. Springer, Cham (2015). https://doi.org/10.1007/978-3-319-26410-3_12
24. Peek, S.T.M., Wouters, E.J.M., van Hoof, J., Luijkx, K.G., Boeije, H.R., Vrijhoef, H.J.M.: Factors influencing acceptance of technology for aging in place: a systematic review. Int. J. Med. Inform. **83**(4), 235–248 (2014)
25. Queirós, A., Silva, A., Alvarelhão, J., Rocha, N.P., Teixeira, A.: Usability, accessibility and ambient-assisted living: a systematic literature review. Univ. Access Inf. Soc. **14**(1), 57–66 (2015)
26. de Ruyter, B., Pelgrim, E.: Ambient assisted-living research in CareLab. Interactions **14**(4), 30–33 (2007)
27. Schomakers, E.M., van Heek, J., Ziefle, M.: A game of wants and needs. The playful, user-centered assessment of AAL technology acceptance. In: ICT4AgeingWell 2018, pp. 126–133 (2018)
28. Silverstone, R., Morley, D., Dahlberg, A., Livingstone, S.: Families, technologies and consumption: the household and information and communication technologies. Technical report (1989)
29. Sixsmith, A., et al.: SOPRANO – an ambient assisted living system for supporting older people at home. In: Mokhtari, M., Khalil, I., Bauchet, J., Zhang, D., Nugent, C. (eds.) ICOST 2009. LNCS, vol. 5597, pp. 233–236. Springer, Heidelberg (2009). https://doi.org/10.1007/978-3-642-02868-7_30
30. Trepte, S., Reinecke, L., Ellison, N.B., Quiring, O., Yao, M.Z., Ziegele, M.: A cross-cultural perspective on the privacy calculus. Soc. Media + Soc. **3**(1), 1–13 (2017)
31. Venkatesh, V., Morris, M.G., Davis, G.B., Davis, F.D.: User acceptance of information technology: toward a unified view. MIS Q. **27**(3), 425–478 (2003)
32. Walker, A., Maltby, T.: Active ageing: a strategic policy solution to demographic ageing in the European Union. Int. J. Soc. Welf. **21**(s1), S117–S130 (2012)
33. Wichert, R., Furfari, F., Kung, A., Tazari, M.R.: How to overcome the market entrance barrier and achieve the market breakthrough in AAL. In: Wichert, R., Eberhardt, B. (eds.) Ambient Assisted Living. ATSC, pp. 349–358. Springer, Heidelberg (2012). https://doi.org/10.1007/978-3-642-27491-6_25
34. Wiles, J.L., Leibing, A., Guberman, N., Reeve, J., Allen, R.E.: The meaning of "aging in place" to older people. Gerontologist **52**(3), 357–366 (2012)
35. Wilkowska, W., Ziefle, M., Himmel, S.: Perceptions of personal privacy in smart home technologies: do user assessments vary depending on the research method? In: Tryfonas, T., Askoxylakis, I. (eds.) HAS 2015. LNCS, vol. 9190, pp. 592–603. Springer, Cham (2015). https://doi.org/10.1007/978-3-319-20376-8_53
36. Xu, H., Dinev, T., Smith, H.J., Hart, P.: Examining the formation of individual's privacy concerns: toward an integrative view. In: International Conference on Information Systems (2008)

Determinants of Trust in Acceptance of Medical Assistive Technologies

Wiktoria Wilkowska[✉] and Martina Ziefle

Human-Computer Interaction Center, RWTH Aachen University,
Campus Boulevard 57, Aachen, Germany
wilkowska@comm.rwth-aachen.de

Abstract. This article examines the relevance of trust in the process of adoption of health-related technologies in home environments. In a multi-method empirical approach this topic is firstly qualitatively explored (focus groups) and in the second step the findings are quantitatively validated (online questionnaire). The research focused on different user factors (user diversity) in the evaluation of opinions and attitudes towards the relevance of trust conditions (e.g., reliability, trustworthiness, operability) and trust "mediators" (e.g., physician as a role model, scientific evidence, hands-on experience) as well as assessment of the importance and expectations regarding various features of the devices. Results showed significant effects of factors age and gender, and influences of persons' health conditions on the examined trust indicators. In addition, analyses revealed that aspects of trust in medical assistive technology to a certain degree can be perceived as predictors of technology acceptance. Next to trust, the findings of this research underline the relevance of considering the users' diversity in the research and design of health-supporting technologies in home environments in order to ensure their successful integration in the long term.

Keywords: Trust · User diversity · Technology acceptance ·
Medical assistive technology

1 Introduction

In the recent years, there is considerable interest in exploiting the potential of innovative advancements in the area of digital technology solutions to enhance the quality and safety of healthcare. Medical assistive technology – also referred to as electronic health technology (eHealth) – in the context of Ambient Assisted Living (AAL) represent one of the biggest shifts in healthcare today, allowing healthcare organizations to change the way healthcare is delivered, and users to reframe their view on how they can maintain their health and well-being more independently. Considering the potential advantages, many stakeholders and institutions make currently efforts to enable and/or improve the infrastructure in this regard to ensure a widespread use of the promising health-supporting technologies at home.

Medical assistive technology devices, which continuously monitor the relevant vital parameters and offer support to manage health-related issues in everyday life (curative) as well as to preserve the well-being of people (preventive) outside of traditional

© Springer Nature Switzerland AG 2019
P. D. Bamidis et al. (Eds.): ICT4AWE 2018, CCIS 982, pp. 45–65, 2019.
https://doi.org/10.1007/978-3-030-15736-4_3

medical institutions, have a great potential to rapidly become common tools to support health-care in people's homes. Despite these promising advantages, the success of the adoption of such ambient medical technologies largely depends on the extent to which users accept, trust in, and can rely on the equipment. In addition, it is crucial to understand how people will trust in such monitoring ambient technology systems while achieving and maintaining their privacy [1]. Especially in the area of health-related technology, it is therefore important to identify special requirements of the (potential) users and adapt the devices to those needs or wishes. To do so, not only focus on a flawless usability of the particular devices, but also a careful examination of the differences between the users and integration of appropriate user-oriented solutions are required.

1.1   The Phenomenon of Trust

Research on the implementation of information systems indicates that trust is an important player in helping users to overcome perceptions of risk and uncertainty in the use and acceptance of technical innovations [2, 3]. Despite the broad consensus about the relevance of technology-related trust in our technology saturated societies [4, 5], the phenomenon of trust is anything but clear and consistent in the relevant literature. It refers not only to the different contexts of the technology applications (e.g., virtual reality, information and communication technologies, intelligent physical environments, e-commerce, etc.) but also to people's trust in a secure digital infrastructure, including sources of information, data, personal assistants, processes and software.

There is an extensive amount of research with respect to trust in technology. However, the different contexts of technology deployment and the various areas to which trust research is connected to leads to a certain fuzziness of its definition, resulting in difficulties to clearly understand and operationalize the term. Another reason for the unsharpness in the definition is, next to the multi-contextual nature, its multidisciplinarity. For instance, Boon and Holmes [6] defined it as "a state involving confident positive expectations about another's motives with respect to oneself in situations entailing risk" (p. 194). Within the field of e-commerce, trust is related to three perceptual factors that have an impact on online trust: perception of credibility, ease of use and risk [7]. Then again, Wang and Emurian [8] identified four elements of online trust regarding interface design features, which relate to graphic, structure, content and social-cue design. Moreover, Siau and Shen [9] provided evidence that the design of an interface can significantly impact the perceived trustworthiness of a system in the field of mobile technologies. Thus, researchers predominantly conceptualize trust according to the features of a particular context [10].

Studies involved in the development of a framework for the construct of trust in health-related technology [11] proved that the trust in medical technology empirically differs from the general trust in other kinds of technology (e.g. information and communication technology, entertainment technology, etc.). The phenomenon of trust seems to be more indispensable when health-relevant aspects are technology-mediated [12]. The concept is multi-layered and includes different components which might be important for understanding how the acceptance and long-term adoption of health-enhancing technologies can be ensured. Personalization, motivation, expertise, familiarity, predictability, sensitivity, and the source of the information are only few such factors that can essentially affect the trust in this regard.

Due to the currently continuously rising number of elderly people which are more prone to frail health, (older) patient's trust in medical technology may be an important factor of functionally working systems; especially since healthcare work systems move to a higher reliance on, and use of, medical technologies [13]. As one of the fundamental attributes in a successful adoption of health-supporting technologies, trust needs to consider a variety of relationships: interpersonal trust (e.g., in the patient-physician communication), trust in environment and infrastructure [5], social trust (e.g., in a healthcare institution) and trust in automation [14].

In the context of emerging AAL solutions, where eHealth technology is meant to daily assist individuals in their habitual environments and support them in terms of their health (e.g., monitoring devices, measurement of vital parameters, sensors recording fall detection, etc.), trust is a particularly important phenomenon, which has been barely researched yet. Persons are confronted with situations, in which they have to trust the medical devices that are incorporated in an ambient technology system and which, depending on how much their health impairments have them rely on this technology, become an inherent part of their life. Also, as health conditions of the users can quickly change, such technology must be highly sensitive, flexible and very adaptive to different circumstances. In this context, trust is more likely to be a dynamic process, which might change depending on the users' characteristics (e.g., age, gender), current health states or their changing life events. Therefore, to understand trust in, and technology acceptance of, health-supportive technologies in home environments not solely flawless operability of the technology is relevant, but also exploration and consideration of differences between the (potential) users is of utmost importance.

1.2 Technology Acceptance

In the present research, we assume that trust is an important component of the medical technology acceptance. Research in this area, originating not only in information systems but also in psychology and sociology, has resulted in several theoretical frameworks. Different user acceptance models have been proposed, examined, refined, extended, and/or unified, providing a good basis for understanding factors and their relationships which influence and facilitate the technology acceptance in users [12]. However, one of the most influential models in this area is the Technology Acceptance Model (TAM) proposed by Davis [15]; the model is depicted in Fig. 1.

TAM was mainly designed for modeling user acceptance in information systems [16]. It represents an instrument to predict the likelihood of the adoption of a new technology and is founded upon the hypothesis that technology acceptance and use can be explained in terms of a user's internal beliefs, attitudes and intentions [17]. The model assumes that an individual's behavioral intention to use a technology is determined by two beliefs: perceived ease of use (extent to which a person believes that using the system would be free of effort) and perceived usefulness (extent to which a person believes that using the system would enhance performance).

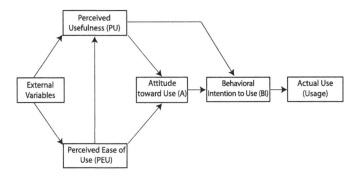

Fig. 1. Technology acceptance model according to Davis [15].

In the present studies, some components of TAM are used as correlates of acceptance of health-supporting ambient systems, examining the influence and predictive power of trust aspects in this regard.

1.3 Differences in Users

For quite some time, scientific research of information technology have perceived that individual differences exert a major force in determining its success [18]. Accordingly, a lot of scientific evidence shows that differences in socio-demographic characteristics (age, gender, education), levels of computer experience, cognitive abilities, attitudes, and personality are significant factors in explaining both technology acceptance and technology user behavior [19–22].

In studies examining users' variability in technology acceptance and performance, especially the factor age plays a relevant role. The findings show that the diversity among the participants of different ages relates not only to the users' belonging to a particular technology generation [23], the connected technology-related know-how and attitudes towards technology (e.g., perceived self-efficacy), but also their mental and physical conditions can vary considerably. All these factors can decisively influence their trust in, and use of, a certain technology system. Therefore, because aging itself is a very complex and differential process, the development of age-sensitive interfaces is on the one side required, but highly challenging on the other side. Similar pattern applies to the users' gender and the resulting differences with respect to technology perceptions and behaviors (e.g., [24–26]). In addition, changes in health conditions and/or unexpected life events can also have a strong impact on the perception of and intention to use medical assistive technology (e.g., [12]).

Recent research dealing with the acceptance of technology in the context of health-supporting technologies in the domestic settings, increasingly considers different users and their specific needs in the development and design process (e.g., [27–30]). However, since this technology is primarily intended for the elderly and people with chronic diseases, it must be also taken into account that their trust in the medical assistive technology may largely differ from the trust of (younger) healthy and carefree users.

1.4 Questions Addressed

Based on the described considerations, the present research contextually explored the concept of trust in the increasingly used medical assistive technology in home environments. The research approach was realized in two empirical studies: First study applied a qualitative research method to explore the topic of trust in the upcoming context from scratch. For this, participants should discuss different trust aspects of the integration of the assistive technology in living environments (socio-technical system) and the trust in a system or institution which manages the health data (social trust), over the interpersonal trust in the communication with the physician in charge through to the perceived reliability and demands regarding technical device or system (technological trust). The results of the first study were validated in a second study, using quantitative method to ensure the generalizability of the findings. Unlike in the previous research in this area, special focus was directed to user diversity which was assumed to considerably influence the trust itself.

2 Method

This article is an extended version of [31] and describes a part of a wider range of studies conducted to explore the users' attitudes as well as perceptions and requirements of medical assistive technology in home environments which is meant to support them in their everyday life both for preventive purposes and to actively monitor their health parameters (for more details see [12]). The concept of these empirical studies uses a user-centered design approach, the main goal of which is to reveal how technical systems must be designed for, and adapted to the individual needs, concepts and mental models of the (potential) users.

In the present study, perceptions of the trust in electronic health technology and users' opinions regarding characteristics that are perceived as necessary for the trusted use of such medical devices, were collected. Moreover, conditions under which the use of such devices is thinkable and additional aspects also perceived as relevant for the user audience were explored and validated. For this purpose, a multi-method empirical approach was pursued which is described in more detail hereafter.

2.1 Multi-method Approach

Considering the user-centered design of the conducted qualitative and quantitative studies, special attention was paid to user diversity (e.g., user's age, gender, physical/health condition, etc.) and the dynamics of personal biographies (e.g., trauma or the onset of an illness). Therefore, some of these criteria were decisive for the composition of the focus groups which represented the first step of the empirical procedure.

Focus Groups. The method of focus groups was chosen as a first step of the empirical study due to its different benefits with respect to the explorative approach. As the group interactions may accentuate members' similarities and differences in a particular context and provide rich information about the range of perspectives, opinions, cognitive beliefs and experiences [32], focus groups were arranged to gather qualitative information about the designated topic. The idea was to explore what people associate with the topic of trust and which aspects are especially relevant for acceptance in the context of using medical assistive devices at home. Therefore, a relevant part – next to the topic of privacy in the context of eHealth technology – were discussions about the aspects which are perceived as important, or even indispensable, for a trustable and accepted (daily) use.

Three differentially compounded focus groups were conducted (N = 15; 60% women), where male and female participants of a wide age range (23–64 years) discussed about their opinions regarding the described topics, answering following questions: "In your opinion, which characteristics of a health-related technology which is used in a home environment are essential?"; and "Which conditions would have to be fulfilled for you to use (and trust) a medical-support device which has to be used at home?". Considering the preceding discussions about the thematically related topics of 'trust' and 'privacy' when dealing with health-supporting equipment, and after the introduction of related topics, like chronic diseases (e.g., cardio-vascular conditions, diabetes, etc.), process of ageing and need for care, the participants presented their requirements, reservations and conditions of usage. In order to increase their acceptance and to assure the long-term adoption, the aim was to find out which basic features of the devices are preconditioned, which other aspects are required by the (potential) users and under which conditions they would trust in, and rely on, interaction with such eHealth devices. The resulting expectations of health-supporting devices which are used in home environments are summarized in Table 1.

Table 1. Expectations for eHealth devices for domestic use (adapted from [31]).

Item description	Scale
– Unconditional reliability	
– Ease of use	
– Low price	
– Seal of approval / test label	
– Attractive / fashionable design	Six-point Likert scale
– Unobtrusiveness	ranging from
– Officially recognized manufacturer	1 = 'not at all important'
– Recommendation of the physician	to 6 = 'very important'
– Financial support of the health insurance for procurement, maintenance, etc.	
– State of the art	
– Strict access control to the health data (e.g., by fingerprint)	

From the methodological point of view, focus group discussions are perfectly suited to gain a deeper insight into the nature of such sensitive and, somehow, difficult-to-grasp topics like the one of trusting in technology, which should support peoples' health. However, there are also restrictions of the method, referring to a comparably small sample size and personally colored results which are unrepresentative. To scientifically ascertain the representativeness of the findings, the outcomes of the focus groups were taken as an empirical base for the subsequent construction of survey items to allow further quantitative data collection with a larger sample.

Quantitative Survey. In the next step of the empirical approach a questionnaire was conducted to quantitatively validate the relevant findings.

The questionnaire included three main parts: In the first part, the respondents answered questions regarding their socio-demographic profiles (e.g., age, gender, professional background, health condition etc.) and reported their experience with health-supporting devices in their daily lives. The second part focused on privacy issues when using the eHealth technology in domestic environments, but this topic will not be further analyzed or discussed in the present paper. The last part of the questionnaire collected data on the trust in the medical assistive technology. To do so, participants (1) assessed the importance of features and characteristics expected/required for the (potentially) used devices, (2) evaluated their degree of approval or rejection on trust-conditions that should be met for accepted usage, and (3) expressed their opinions about complementary statements, retrieved from the focus group discussions, about what else makes the medical technology at home trustworthily.

The participants were recruited through advertisements in local newspapers, social networks on the Internet and collaboration with targeted societal groups (e.g., retirement home). Some of the respondents were also reached through the authors' personal contacts. There was an online version and a paper-based version of the questionnaire (from the latter especially the older participants benefited). On average, it took 15–20 min to complete the questionnaire and the data collection lasted for about four weeks.

2.2 Research Approach

Based on the concept of the user-centered design (e.g., [33, 34]), the research variables focus on different users' factors and their health biographies on the one side, as well as on their expectations and requirements for trusted health-supporting equipment at home, on the other.

Independent Variables. The diversity among the users of technology is huge. They differ not only in their socio-demographic characteristics, but also in their sensory and cognitive skills, physical and motoric capabilities, and various requirements, like those linked to aging, which complicate an easy-going access and interaction with modern technical solutions [12]. To deepen the understanding of this diversity among (potential) eHealth users, and to get insights in their different needs, requirements and wants regarding trust in such a technology, it is crucial to consider different points of view. In the present statistical analyses, we consider, therefore, three independent variables, referring to the participants' diversity:

- *Age* [young (≤ 44 years; 50%) vs. middle-aged and older (45 years and older; 50%)];
- *Gender* [women (46%) vs. men (54%)];
- Perception of the own *health condition* [good (44%) vs. moderate (46%) vs. poor (10%)].

Dependent Variables. The dependent variables of this study refer to the indicators of perceived trust in eHealth technologies, which are used in people's home environments for health monitoring, prevention and rehabilitation. First, the required *features and characteristics* for eHealth devices (see Table 1) are considered as dependent variables. In addition, the *conditions of trust* regarding health-supporting technology in domestic settings are examined. The items were evaluated using a six-point Likert scale ranging from 1 (='strongly disagree') to 6 (='strongly agree'). For a better overview, thematically related aspects are merged into categories as presented in Table 2 (top). Next to the device's reliability which represents the probably most important claim of medical assistive technologies and, hence, builds an unattached category, three other main categories of trust conditions were generated (the internal consistency of the particular categories is indicated between brackets):

- Trustworthiness (Cronbach's alpha α = .71; min = 3, max = 18);
- Operability (Cronbach's alpha α = .73; min = 3, max = 18);
- Easing of the burden of the disease (Cronbach's alpha α = .83; min = 2, max = 12).

Table 2. Conditions (top) and mediators of trust (bottom) in eHealth technology.

	Category / Short description	Item descriptions
Trust Conditions		"I would trust the medical device if...
	Reliability	…it would immediately provide feedback about incorrect information and asks me to repeat the measurement."
	Trust-worthiness	…I would know that it comes from an approved and trustworthy manufacturer."
		…its reliability would be confirmed by a recognized testing institution."
		…I would rarely have to see the doctor thanks to the device."
	Operability	…I would intuitively understand how to handle the device."
		…I would be able to count on customer service in case I experience difficulties."
		…it would allow me to take it anywhere to make measurements."
	Easing	…it would be integrated in my daily life so that I feel relieved from my illness."
		…it would give me the feeling of independence despite my illness."
Trust Mediators	*Doctor as a role model*	"If my doctor relies on medical technology, I trust it."
	Scientific evidence	"I consider medical devices whose quality and functionality are confirmed by scientific studies to be trustworthy."
	Hands-on experience	"I consider medical equipment, which functionality I can try out for a while without paying, to be trustworthy."
	Exchange with peers	"My trust in medical devices would be greater if I could exchange with peers."

Moreover, four *additional statements* (trust "mediators") on what else makes the use of a health-supporting technology at home trustworthy were added as dependent variables. Likewise, participants expressed their level of agreement (6 = 'strongly agree') or disapproval (1 = 'strongly disagree') regarding the aspects presented in the bottom part of Table 2.

2.3 Participants

The random sample intended to cover different population groups including male and female participants in different ages (young, middle-aged and older) and various health conditions, as well as persons with different professional backgrounds and levels of experience with technology.

In total N = 104 persons aged between 21 and 98 years participated in this study (58% women; 42% men). More than 40% of the respondents reported to suffer from chronic health conditions (e.g., cardiovascular diseases, diabetes mellitus, asthma). Overall, more than half of them reported to use health-supporting devices in everyday life: most participants used blood pressure meters (32%), followed by those who used blood sugar meters (10%) and 9% used heart rate monitors; a few (6%) also reported to use hearing aids and insulin pumps.

The participants represented different professions (including teachers, engineers, economists, psychologists and mechanics) and different educational levels. However, the average level of education in the sample was quite high. The participation in the study was voluntary and respondents were not compensated for participating.

3 Results

For statistical analyses, calculating the influence of user diversity on trust in eHealth technology, multiple analyses of variance (MANOVA) were executed and the significance of omnibus F-Tests was taken from Pillai values. For descriptive analyses, the means (M) and standard deviations (SD) are reported, and the parameter partial eta squared (η^2) was calculated for the effect sizes according to Cohen [35]. For the identification of the strongest predictors of the presented trust variables, stepwise multiple regression analysis was performed. The level of statistical significance (p) was set at the conventional 5%.

3.1 Trust Expectations for eHealth Technology

In the first step, the influence of independent variables on the expected trust characteristics is statistically examined. A multivariate analysis of variance revealed a significant omnibus effect of age [$F(11, 76) = 2.1$, $p = 0.033$; $\eta^2 = .23$] and gender [$F(11, 76) = 2.6$, $p = 0.007$; $\eta^2 = .27$].

The effects of age on the between-subject level resulted for the following characteristics: ease of use [$F(1, 98) = 7.6$, $p = 0.007$; $\eta^2 = .08$], low price [$F(1, 98) = 5.9$, $p = 0.017$; $\eta^2 = .06$], officially recognized manufacturer [$F(1, 98) = 7.3$, $p = 0.008$;

$\eta^2 = .08$] and the state of the art [$F(1, 98) = 6.9$, $p = 0.01$; $\eta^2 = .07$]. The resulting means are depicted in Fig. 2. It is evident that the middle-aged and older participants expect significantly higher standards for medical equipment in domestic settings than the young participants.

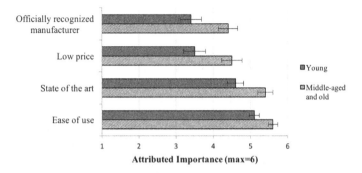

Fig. 2. Effect of age on expectations for eHealth technology in home environments (adapted from [31]).

Considering the impact of gender the on expectations, the particular effects on the between-subject level result for unconditional reliability [$F(1, 98) = 4.6$, $p = 0.035$; $\eta^2 = .05$], seal of approval [$F(1, 98) = 7.7$, $p = 0.007$; $\eta^2 = .08$], ease of use [$F(1, 98) = 20.1$, $p \leq 0.001$; $\eta^2 = .19$] and recommendation of physician [$F(1, 98) = 5.6$, $p = 0.021$; $\eta^2 = .06$]. Descriptive data (Fig. 3) demonstrate that women have higher expectations regarding health-supporting devices than men. According to the effect sizes, the impact of gender is especially meaningful for the ease of use of the medical technology.

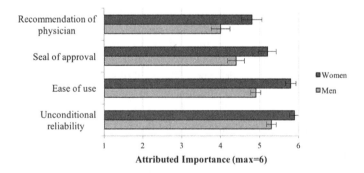

Fig. 3. Effect of gender on expectations for eHealth technology in home environments (adapted from [31]).

3.2 Trust Conditions for eHealth Technology

The influence of the user diversity on the conditions of use of health-supporting technologies in domestic settings were examined in the next step.

An ANOVA revealed a significant main effect of gender on the condition of flawless operability of the digital medical technology [$F(1, 101) = 4.2$, $p = 0.043$; $\eta^2 = .04$] which is depicted in Fig. 4 (right): Women demand evidently higher standards ($M = 15.1$, $SD = 2.8$) with regard to the intuitive, service-related and location-independent eHealth technology in comparison to men ($M = 13.5$, $SD = 3$).

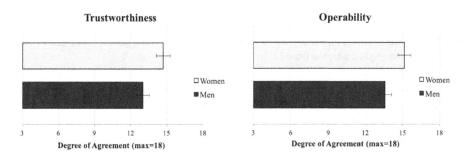

Fig. 4. Main effect of gender on the conditions of operability (left) and trustworthiness (right) when using eHealth technology in home environments (adapted from [31]).

A similar pattern is noticeable considering the conditions that form the category of trustworthiness [$F(1, 100) = 4.4$, $p = 0.039$; partial $\eta^2 = .05$]. The mean values are showed on the left in Fig. 4 (women: $M = 14.7$, $SD = 3$; men: $M = 13$, $SD = 3.4$). Even when, according to the rather small effect sizes, the impact of gender is minor in both cases, the results indicate that women demand more stringent conditions for medical equipment than men.

In addition to these main effects, the univariate ANOVA revealed moderate interacting effects of age and gender [$F(1, 100) = 8.7$, $p = 0.004$; partial $\eta^2 = .09$], as well as of gender and perceived health conditions [$F(2, 100) = 4.4$, $p = 0.014$; partial $\eta^2 = .09$], on the trustworthiness in health-supporting technology. Especially in the younger age group, men ($M = 11.1$, $SD = 0.8$) and women ($M = 15.1$, $SD = 0.8$) differ significantly, whereby women demand higher standards of trustworthiness in this context. As opposed to this, the differences in the group of middle-aged and older participants are not so evident between women ($M = 14.3$, $SD = 0.8$) and men ($M = 15$, $SD = 0.7$). The interaction is presented on the left in Fig. 5. Figure 5 at the right side depicts also that the additional influence of health condition especially splits the opinions of those who report bad health: Whereas women require very high standards of trustworthiness ($M = 16$, $SD = 1.5$), men with poor health do not pay as much attention to this condition ($M = 10.1$, $SD = 1.3$). On the contrary, in the groups of good and moderate health both genders do not significantly differ in their opinions, both reaching high means for the condition of trustworthiness.

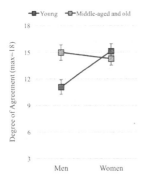
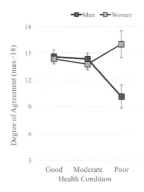

Fig. 5. Interaction effects on the conditions of trustworthiness: age and gender (left), gender and health condition (right); adapted from [31].

Moreover, statistical analyses of the trust conditions of reliability and of the easing of the burden of the disease, yielded no significant influences of any of the user diversity variables. According to this finding, all participants – independently from the analyzed users' factors – wished for highly reliable medical equipment which serves the purpose of exoneration.

3.3 Trust 'Mediators' for eHealth Technology

The remaining items, resulting from the aforementioned group discussions (see Table 2 bottom), complete the analyses and were considered as trust 'mediators' for the use of medical technology. The technique of three-way analysis of variance was chosen for the statistical evaluation.

Considering the aspect *'doctor as a role model'* as relevant for the trust in medical devices, an ANOVA with the factors age, gender and health condition revealed a significant effect of the participants' age [$F(1, 102) = 4.1$, $p = 0.046$; $\eta^2 = .04$]. In Fig. 6 differences between the means reached for both age groups are depicted. Even if the differences in the perceptions are small, the outcome shows that persons aged 45 years and older ($M = 3.6$, $SD = 1.5$) confide in the opinion of the doctor, who relies on the assistive technology, more than the younger people ($M = 4.2$, $SD = 1.5$).

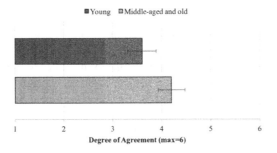

Fig. 6. Main effect of age on the trust aspect 'doctor as a role model' for using eHealth technology at home (adapted from [31]).

In addition, for the aspect of *'scientific evidence'* the analysis of variance showed a moderate and strong influence of the user factors: (1) main effect of age [$F(1, 101) = 6.1$, $p = 0.015$; $\eta^2 = .06$]; (2) main effect of gender [$F(1, 101) = 4.5, p = 0.036$; $\eta^2 = .05$]; and (3) an interacting effect of gender and health condition [$F(1, 101) = 6.1, p = 0.003$; $\eta^2 = .12$]. The moderate effect of age (Fig. 7, left) shows that middle-aged and older people ($M = 4.9, SD = 1.2$) perceive medical devices whose quality and functionality is confirmed by scientific studies as more trustworthy than the younger participants ($M = 4.1, SD = 1.4$). Regarding the influence of gender (on the right in Fig. 7), women's average values ($M = 4.9, SD = 1.2$) exceed those of men ($M = 4.1, SD = 1.5$), meaning that women's trust in medical equipment at home is slightly more shaped by scientific studies.

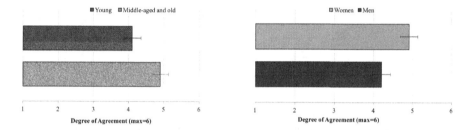

Fig. 7. Main effects of age (left) and gender (right) on the trust aspect 'scientific evidence' for using eHealth technology at home (adapted from [31]).

Besides, an interacting effect of gender and the perceived health condition resulted for the aspect of 'scientific evidence'; The mean values of the particular groups are presented in Fig. 8. Interestingly, for both genders the biggest differences result for those who report poor health conditions, and women with poor health ($M = 5.7$, $SD = 0.5$) attach significantly higher importance to scientific evidence than men with the same health status ($M = 3, SD = 2$).

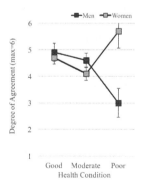

Fig. 8. Interacting effect of gender and health condition on the trust aspect 'scientific evidence' for using eHealth technology at home (adapted from [31]).

A significant interaction effect of gender and health condition results additionally for the trust aspect of '*exchange with peers*' [$F(2, 102) = 4.3$, $p = 0.016$; $\eta^2 = .09$]. The pattern is similar to the previous analysis: Compared to persons with good and moderate health in both genders, the opinions diverge for men and women with poor health conditions. Thereby, women ($M = 5$, $SD = 0.8$) consider it to be more important to exchange their opinions with peers than men ($M = 2.9$, $SD = 1.6$). The interaction effect is showed in Fig. 9.

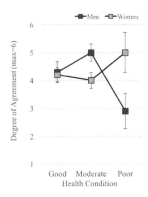

Fig. 9. Interacting effect of gender and health condition on the trust aspect 'exchange with peers' for using eHealth technology at home (adapted from [31]).

For the aspect of '*hands-on experience*' the results are neither age-, gender-, nor health status-specific.

3.4 Trust Predictors for the Acceptance of eHealth Technology

In addition to the impact of user diversity on the researched trust variables, it is of great interest which of the discussed trust criteria represent the best predictors for a successful long-term adoption of the medical technology in private living spaces.

For this purpose, in the last step of the statistical computing two acceptance correlates, based on Technology Acceptance Model [15], are analyzed in a stepwise multiple regression calculations: perceived usefulness ("In your opinion, how useful are medical assistive technology devices in private environments?") and intention to use ("I'm willing to invest in and use useful medical technology."). The regression models resulting from the analysis of all trust-variables are given in Table 3 and the findings are discussed below.

Table 3. Results of the multiple regression analysis for the adoption of eHealth in home environments (***p ≤ .001, **p ≤ .01, *p ≤ .05; VIF = variance inflation factor < 10).

Predictors		R^2	β	t	VIF	ANOVA
Perceived Usefulness	Operability	14.5%	.32	3.2**	1.0	F(2,92)=7.6, p≤.001
	Scientific evidence		.23	2.1*	1.25	
Intention to use eHealth	Trustworthiness	32.9%	-.12	-1.1	1.0	F(4,94)=11, p≤.001
	Scientific evidence		.39	3.7***	1.07	
	Hands-on experience		.24	2.2*	1.09	
	Officially recognized manufacturer		.21	2.2*	1.12	

The prediction model for the perceived usefulness of health-supporting technology in home environments contained two predictors. The model was statistically significant, $F(2, 92) = 7.6$, $p \leq .001$, and accounted for approximately 15 percent of the variance of the perceived usefulness (adjusted $R^2 = .126$). The variable flawless operability received the strongest weight in this model ($\beta = .32$) making its unique contribution to explain the dependent variable and was followed by the relevance of scientific evidence ($\beta = .23$). Thus, for this model, operability [$t(92) = 3.2, p = 0.002$] and scientific evidence [$t(92) = 2.1$, $p = 0.036$] are the significant predictors of the acceptance (= perceived usefulness) of health-supportive ambient technology. From the top part of Table 3 it is evident that the values of the variance inflation factor are well below 10; additionally, the tolerance statistics are well above 0.2 which confirms no collinearity within the presented data. From the regression model it results the following linear equation:

$$Perceived\ usefulness = 2.6 + 0.6(operability) + 0.14(scientific\ evidence) \quad (1)$$

For the intention to use eHealth technology in home environment, the regression model contained four predictors, including a condition of trust, two trust 'mediators' and an expected feature of the devices as summarized in the bottom part of Table 3. The model reaches statistical significance [$F(4, 94) = 11$, p $\leq$ .001] and explains overall almost 33 % of the variance regarding the acceptability indicator of eHealth technology (adjusted $R^2 = .300$). As the strongest predictor for the intention to use emerged the scientific evidence ($\beta = .39$; $t(95) = 3.7, p \leq 0.001$), followed by hands-on experience ($\beta = .24$; $t(95) = 2.2$, $p = 0.031$), the expectation of an officially recognized manufacturer ($\beta = .21$; $t(95) = 2.2, p = 0.028$) and trustworthiness ($\beta = -.12$; $t(95) = -1.1$, n.s.). The VIF and tolerance values suggest no collinearity within the present data. The resulting equation for intention to use eHealth is presented below:

$$Intention\ to\ use = 1.6 + 0.39(scientific\ evidence) + 0.24(hands\text{-}on\ experience)$$
$$+\ 0.19(officially\ recognized\ manufacturer) - 0.5(trustworthiness) \quad (2)$$

According to the presented findings for both indicators of technology acceptance, trust aspects can partly predict how successful the ambient technology will be. Hence, it is a clear evidence that the evaluated factors – even if certainly not the only decisive – are relevant for the acceptance and, therefore, for the long-term integration of health-supportive technologies in the domestic settings.

4 Discussion and Future Research Outline

Patients' trust is an inevitable component of the future development and design of medical innovations that are increasingly implemented in home environments. Health and disease are inherent parts of humankind which directly affect people's well-being, personal identity formation and life-span development. Therefore, any technology that seeks to be supportive for medical treatment and care needs to consider highly sensitive social and individual issues, regarding both physical and mental conditions.

However, trust is a complex phenomenon [11, 31, 36], which is determined by many aspects: It depends on individual coping strategies with regard to illness, and persons' affective and cognitive characteristics (e.g., risk taking behavior, technical self-confidence), their experience with technical devices as well as their self-efficacy when using technology, in general, and medical technology, in particular. In addition, the extent of trust and the trustfulness might also be shaped by the respective usage context and in dependence on the onset of an illness. Thus, trust in medical technologies might vary even within one user, for instance in times of essential and vital using conditions in comparison to those situations in which medical technology assistance is important, however, neither time-critical nor decisive.

In this research, we empirically explored the understanding of potential users of trust in, and trustworthiness of, medical technology which is predominately used in home environments. Especially in the context of aging societies, it is a crucial question, how trust in health-related technologies is formed and how it can be supported. It is challenging to predict how older adults react when it comes to the use of medical technology and which trust requirements they form in this context. One could speculate that especially the group of older and life-experienced people might be less sensitive in terms of technology acceptance and shows a higher trust, since they, due to the health issues, typically have no choice but to use such equipment in order to meet the daily life requirements. On the other hand, it is also possible that older adults show only limited trust attitudes as they usually have a lower experience with technology use, and, as a consequence, a lower self-confidence with technical devices.

To empirically address these questions, we pursued a two-step research procedure (qualitative and quantitative method) and invited users of different ages, of both genders and with different health conditions to share their opinions and attitudes towards the importance of trust "determinants" (as, e.g., reliability, trustworthiness, operability and easing) and trust "mediators" (doctor as a role model, scientific evidence, exchange with peers and hands-on experience). Also, we analyzed the relevance of different system features.

4.1   Major Outcomes and Classification of the Results

Overall, we found both findings, which show an impact of user diversity on trust in medical technologies, and findings, which hint at a quite homogeneous picture.

With respect to the gender effects, it was found that women attached a higher importance to the ease of using medical technology in comparison to male users. Women also reported to rely their trust in eHealth technology on scientific evidence as an external quality validation. In addition, female users with a poor health condition indicated higher relevance of the exchange with peers, while in the opinion of men such an exchange is not that important for trustworthiness.

Regarding the age effects, older persons attach more importance to opinions of doctors and medical stuff, and wish higher standards for medical equipment compared to younger users. However, there are also user diversity-insensitive attitudes: outcomes with respect to the required trust conditions of reliability and the easing of the burden of the disease yielded no significant influences of age, gender, or health condition.

Taking a more general perspective, it is of great importance that the technical design especially in the field of medical technology is aligned with the demands of the respective end users, their requirements in terms of social usage, and their needs for dignity and individualism. Beyond functional and medical requirements, thus, acceptance and usability in line with intimacy and trust cognitions should be a benchmark for the design of a socially responsible medical technology.

4.2   Research Directions and Limitations

Even when valuable insights into the perceptions of trust and trustworthiness in the context of use of eHealth technologies in home environments could be gained, the phenomenon of trust still remains highly complex. The presented empirical approach has some limitations which should be considered and relevant research directions should be outlined.

Relevant Attributes Under Study. In this research, the spectrum of the examined trust-relevant attributes is obviously limited, as the presented studies represent only a first step in this regard. Naturally, there are many more aspects which require a closer analysis in future work. The same applies to the impact of demographic variables on the perceptions of trust. So far, we only looked in a quite rough analysis for age and gender effects. From the perspective of a social science, however, age and gender are complex factors which are assumed to be carriers for social roles, upbringing, societal attitudes, life experience, domain knowledge, skills and expertise, and general wisdom [37]. Thus, those factors should be analyzed in relation to age and gender to gain deeper insights. Especially when it comes to age and aging, it is important to refer to different values on, and perspectives of, culturally and societally anchored aging concepts [38, 39]. Because, the moment users feel old, and the moment they are old might largely differ, depending on individual perspectives, but also on cultural and economic dimensions [40–42].

Cultural Diversity. Even though the sample size might be methodologically and statistically appropriate for the carried-out analyses, it is still apparent that trust in health-relevant technology use is inevitably intermingled with lifelong-learning and the understanding of broader user groups and cultural diversity. In many cultures being old and ill is perceived as a stigma [37] and is directly related to ageism—the negative societal framing of age and aging which is difficult to accept. Moreover, the combination of old age and chronic disease is closely related to the end-of-life emotions, which are personality issues the patients are highly sensitive to; however, these also depend on different coping strategies and the way of framing by societal and cultural values [43]. Future studies should, therefore, focus on more aspects of trust, additionally addressing the understanding of trust in an intercultural setting.

Governance and Policy. We should be also aware that the trust in medical technology and care has a policy component [44]. In this context, it should be examined if the perceptions of trust and trustworthiness meet an appropriate competence of the medical treatments and education of medical professionals on the one hand, as well as the individuals' confidence in the national or international efforts for ethical human care and the diversity-fair treatment of patients at an older age, on the other hand [45].

4.3   Future Research Lines

Referring to the latter, in the research of trust of medical assistive technologies future research lines should direct to some important topics, which need to be considered in line with a responsible research and innovation policy [46, 47]. The most important focal points in the context of using eHealth technologies in private homes are listed below.

Big Data and Privacy Issues. In times of big data and the emerging relevance of the transportation and storage of medical/health data, electronic services and medical technology evolve into an enormous marketing good which contributes to the gain of knowledge, on the one, and marketing success, on the other hand [48, 49]. The decision to share private medical data is therefore a delicate question for patients, who need to weigh up between sharing their health-related data (and thereby support the societal medical gain of knowledge) and hiding their personal data and, thus, preserve their privacy and personal identity [50, 51].

Age, Aging and Ageism. Individual and societal values of aging are formed by cultures and socialization in line with economic, political and societal changes. Therefore, trust in a technology that supports care depends on the societal framing of the value of aging and the consideration of life-span developments [42]. Thus, the acceptance patterns of, and trust in, medical care need to be also analyzed against the background of culture, culturally-formed trade-offs between societally acknowledged caring mission of the very old, and the aspect of their life-end decisions [52].

Frailness, Functional Independence and Course of Disease. The openness to trust and accept eHealth technology necessarily depends on the health status. In this context, it might be essential to consider different types of disease and etiopathologies. Especially patients who suffer from chronic and serious diseases need to cope with the severity of the illness, the frailness and the end-of-life cognitions in a much deeper and complex manner than patients with a temporary need for the assistance of medical equipment.

Different Perspectives of Stakeholders. So far, research regarding the trust in medical technology mostly considers the perspective of patients [11, 12, 29]. However, the entire caring situation as well as the different people participating and their roles which support the nursing care, are also of paramount importance and need to be mandatory integrated in the concept of trust towards medical technology and treatment.

Acknowledgements. The authors thank all participants for their patience and openness to share opinions on trust in medical technology. This work has been funded partly by Excellence Initiative of Germany's Federal Ministry of Education and Research and the German Research Foundation and partly by the project PAAL, funded by the German Ministry of Research and Education (under the reference number 6SV7955).

References

1. Little, L., Marsh, S., Briggs, P.: Trust and privacy permissions for an ambient world. In: Trust in e-Services: Technologies, Practices and Challenges, pp. 259–292. IGI Global, Hershey (2007)
2. Li, X., Hess, T.J., Valacich, J.S.: Why do we trust new technology? A study of initial trust formation with organizational information systems. J. Strateg. Inf. Syst. **17**(1), 39–71 (2008)
3. Pavlou, P.A., Gefen, D.: Building effective online marketplaces with institution-based trust. Inf. Syst. Res. **15**(1), 37–59 (2004)
4. Lewis, J.D., Weigert, A.: Trust as a social reality. Soc. Forces **63**(4), 967–985 (1985)
5. Falcone, R., Castelfranchi, C.: The socio-cognitive dynamics of trust: does trust create trust? Trust Cyber-Soc. **2246**, 55–72 (2001)
6. Boon, S.D., Holmes, J.G.: Cooperation and Prosocial Behaviour, 1st edn. Cambridge University Press, Cambridge (1991)
7. Corritore, C.L., Kracher, B., Wiedenbeck, S.: Online trust: concepts, evolving themes, a model. Int. J. Hum. Comput. Stud. **58**(6), 737–758 (2003)
8. Wang, Y.D., Emurain, H.H.: An overview of online trust: concepts, elements and implications. Comput. Hum. Behav. **21**, 105–125 (2005)
9. Siau, K., Shen, Z.: Building customer trust in mobile commerce. Commun. ACM **46**(4), 91–94 (2003)
10. Sillence, E., Briggs, P., Harris, P., Fishwick, L.: A framework for understanding trust factors in web-based health advice. Int. J. Hum.0 Comput. Stud. **64**(8), 697–713 (2006)
11. Montague, E.N., Kleiner, B.M., Winchester, W.W.: Empirically understanding trust in medical technology. Int. J. Ind. Ergon. **39**(4), 628–634 (2009)
12. Wilkowska, W.: Acceptance of eHealth Technology in Home Environments: Advanced Studies on User Diversity in Ambient Assisted Living. Apprimus, Aachen (2015)
13. Montague, E.N.: Validation of a trust in medical technology instrument. Appl. Ergon. **41**(6), 812–821 (2010)
14. Muir, B.: Trust in automation: part 1. Theoretical issues in the study and human intervention in automated systems. Ergonomics **37**, 1905–1923 (1994)
15. Davis, F.D.: Perceived usefulness, perceived ease of use, and user acceptance of information technology. MIS Q. **13**(3), 319–340 (1989)
16. Mathieson, K., Peacock, E., Chin, W.W.: Extending the technology acceptance model: the influence of perceived user resources. ACM SIGMIS Database **32**(3), 86–112 (2001)

17. Turner, M., Kitchenham, B., Brereton, P., Charters, S., Budgen, D.: Does the technology acceptance model predict actual use? A systematic literature review. Inf. Softw. Technol. **52** (5), 463–479 (2010)
18. Zmud, R.W.: Individual differences and MIS success: a review of the empirical literature. Manag. Sci. **25**(10), 966–979 (1979)
19. Gefen, D., Straub, D.W.: Gender differences in the perception and use of e-mail: an extension to the technology acceptance model. MIS Q. **21**(4), 389–400 (1997)
20. Rogers, W.A., Fisk, A.D.: Human Factors, Applied Cognition, and Aging. Lawrence Erlbaum Associates Publishers, Mahwah (2000)
21. Ong, C.-S., Lai, J.-Y.: Gender differences in perceptions and relation-ships among dominants of e-learning acceptance. Comput. Hum. Behav. **22**(5), 816–829 (2006)
22. Wilkowska, W., Ziefle, M.: Which factors form older adults' acceptance of mobile information and communication technologies? In: Holzinger, A., Miesenberger, K. (eds.) USAB 2009. LNCS, vol. 5889, pp. 81–101. Springer, Heidelberg (2009). https://doi.org/10. 1007/978-3-642-10308-7_6
23. Sackmann, R., Winkler, O.: Technology generations revisited: the internet generation. Gerontechnology **11**(4), 493–503 (2013)
24. Schumacher, P., Morahan-Martin, J.: Gender, internet and computer attitudes and experiences. Comput. Hum. Behav. **17**(1), 95–110 (2001)
25. Broos, A.: Gender and information and communication technologies (ICT) anxiety: male self-assurance and female hesitation. Cyber Psychol. Behav. **8**(1), 21–31 (2005)
26. Kowalewski, S., Wilkowska, W., Ziefle, M.: Accounting for user diversity in the acceptance of medical assistive technologies. In: Szomszor, M., Kostkova, P. (eds.) eHealth 2010. LNICST, vol. 69, pp. 175–183. Springer, Heidelberg (2011). https://doi.org/10.1007/978-3-642-23635-8_22
27. Demiris, G., et al.: Older adults' attitudes towards and perceptions of 'smart home' technologies: a pilot study. Med. Inform. Internet Med. **29**(2), 87–94 (2004)
28. Klack, L., Schmitz-Rode, T., Wilkowska, W., Kasugai, K., Heidrich, F., Ziefle, M.: Integrated home monitoring and compliance optimization for patients with mechanical circulatory support devices. Ann. Biomed. Eng. **39**(12), 2911–2921 (2011)
29. Wilkowska, W., Ziefle, M.: User diversity as a challenge for the integration of medical technology into future smart home environments. In: Human-Centered Design of E-Health Technologies, pp. 95–126. Hershey, PA (2011)
30. Ziefle, M., Brauner, P., van Heek, J.: Intentions to use smart textiles in AAL home environments: comparing younger and older adults. In: Zhou, J., Salvendy, G. (eds.) ITAP 2016. LNCS, vol. 9754, pp. 266–276. Springer, Cham (2016). https://doi.org/10.1007/978-3-319-39943-0_26
31. Wilkowska, W., Ziefle, M.: Understanding trust in medical technologies. In: Proceedings of the 4th International Conference on Communication and Information Technologies for Ageing Well and e-Health (ICT4AWE 2018), pp. 62–73. SCITEPRESS (2018)
32. Lambert, S.D., Loiselle, C.G.: Combining individual interviews and focus groups to enhance data richness. J. Adv. Nurs. **62**(2), 228–237 (2008)
33. Abras, C., Maloney-Krichmar, D., Preece, J.: User-centered design. In: Bainbridge, W. (ed.) Encyclopedia of Human-Computer Interaction, vol. 37, no. 4, pp. 445–456. Sage Publications, Thousand Oaks (2004)
34. Mao, J.Y., Vredenburg, K., Smith, P.W., Carey, T.: The state of user-centered design practice. Commun. ACM **48**(3), 105–109 (2005)
35. Cohen, J.: Statistical Power Analysis for the Behavioral Sciences. Erlbaum, Hillsdale (1988)

36. Ziefle, M., Röcker, C., Holzinger, A.: Medical technology in smart homes: exploring the user's perspective on privacy, intimacy and trust. In: IEEE 35th Annual Computer Software and Applications Conference Workshops (COMPSACW), pp. 410–415 (2011)
37. Ziefle, M., Schaar, A.K.: Gender differences in acceptance and attitudes towards an invasive medical stent. Electron. J. Health Inform. **6**(2), e13 (2011)
38. Moody, H.R.: Aging: Concepts and Controversies. Pine Forge Press, Newbury Park (2006)
39. Morrow-Howell, N., Hinterlong, J., Sherraden, M.: Productive Aging: Concepts and Challenges. JHU Press, Baltimore (2001)
40. Thiede, M.: Information and access to health care: is there a role for trust? Soc. Sci. Med. **61**(7), 1452–1462 (2005)
41. Hallenbeck, J.L.: Intercultural differences and communication at the end of life. Prim. Care: Clin. Office Pract. **28**(2), 401–413 (2001)
42. Resnick, B., Gwyther, L.P., Roberto, K.A.: Resilience in Aging: Concepts, Research, and Outcomes. Springer, New York (2010). https://doi.org/10.1007/978-1-4419-0232-0
43. Hamel, L., Wu, B., Brodie, M.: Views and experiences with end-of-life medical care in the US [Internet]. Kaiser Family Foundation (2017)
44. Mechanic, D.: The functions and limitations of trust in the provision of medical care. J. Health Polit. Policy Law **23**(4), 661–686 (1998)
45. Wilkowska, W., Brauner, P., Ziefle, M.: Rethinking Technology development for older adults. A responsible research and innovation duty. In: Aging, Technology, and Health. Elsevier North Holland, Amsterdam (2018)
46. Stahl, B.C.: Responsible research and innovation: the role of privacy in an emerging framework. Sci. Publ. Policy **40**(6), 708–716 (2013)
47. Stahl, B.C., Eden, G., Jirotka, M.: Responsible research and innovation in information and communication technology: Identifying and engaging with the ethical implications of ICTs. In: Responsible Innovation, pp. 199–218 (2013)
48. Vervier, L., Zeissig, E.M., Lidynia, C., Ziefle, M.: Perceptions of digital footprints and the value of privacy. In: Proceedings of the International Conference on Internet of Things and Big Data (IoTBD 2017), pp. 80–91. SCITEPRESS (2017)
49. van Heek, J., Himmel, S., Ziefle, M.: Caregivers' perspectives on ambient assisted living technologies in professional care contexts. In: 4th International Conference on Information and Communication Technologies for Ageing Well and e-Health (ICT4AWE 2018), pp. 37–48. SCITEPRESS (2018)
50. Calero Valdez, A., Ziefle, M.: The users' perspective on privacy trade-offs in health recommender systems. Int. J. Hum.-Comput. Stud. **121**, 108–121 (2019)
51. Ziefle, M., Halbey, J., Kowalewski, S.: Users' willingness to share data in the internet: perceived benefits and caveats. In: Proceedings of the International Conference on Internet of Things and Big Data (IoTBD 2016), pp. 255–265. SCITEPRESS (2016)
52. Bowling, A., Banister, D., Sutton, S., Evans, O., Windsor, J.: A multidimensional model of the quality of life in older age. Aging Ment. Health **6**(4), 355–371 (2002)

The Best of Both Worlds: Combining Digital and Human AAL Advisory Services for Older Adults

Diotima Bertel[1(✉)], Soraia Teles[2,3], Flora Strohmeier[1],
Pedro Vieira-Marques[3], Paul Schmitter[4], Stefan H. Ruscher[1],
Constança Paúl[2,3], and Andrea Ch. Kofler[4]

[1] Research and Development Department, SYNYO GmbH,
Otto-Bauer-Gasse 5/14, 1060 Vienna, Austria
diotima.bertel@synyo.com,
flora.strohmeier@gmail.com, stefanh.ruscher@gmail.com
[2] Department of Behavioral Sciences,
Institute of Biomedical Sciences Abel Salazar (ICBAS),
University of Porto, Rua de Jorge Viterbo Ferreira, 228,
4050-313 Porto, Portugal
teles.s.soraia@gmail.com, paul@icbas.up.pt
[3] Center for Health Technology and Services Research (CINTESIS),
University of Porto, Rua Dr. Plácido Da Costa, 4200-450 Porto, Portugal
pmarques@med.up.pt
[4] Zurich University of Applied Sciences,
Grüental, 8820 Wädenswil, Zurich, Switzerland
{paul.schmitter,andrea.kofler}@zhaw.ch

Abstract. Technological developments in the last 20 years have been instrumental in service provision by offering new means of interaction among stakeholders in virtual environments. However, in most service sectors, the consumer journey is growing in complexity, which calls for a multifaceted service logic. While a number of ICT companies have been expanding their portfolio from an entirely virtual to additional physical experience, a seamless merger of both physical and virtual worlds in service provision may still be some way off. This applies to advisory services for Ambient Assisted Living (AAL) solutions, a recently opened market of great importance in the contemporary ageing society. In this position paper, we expand on the concepts of engagement platforms and engagement ecosystems to argue that an integration of physical and virtual worlds is necessary for AAL advisory services. We first determine the extent to which current service platforms are acting as 'engagement platforms' by presenting key insights from an analysis of platforms and services promoting AAL products for older adults. The focus lays on the stakeholder involvement, the interaction and feedback features. Second, we identify the key features that a platform must have to qualify as an engagement platform. Third, the debate delves deeper on how to integrate both virtual and physical dimensions in an optimal solution for stakeholders' engagement. Finally, we present the concept of an 'Authorized Active Advisor' as a solution

© Springer Nature Switzerland AG 2019
P. D. Bamidis et al. (Eds.): ICT4AWE 2018, CCIS 982, pp. 66–82, 2019.
https://doi.org/10.1007/978-3-030-15736-4_4

of utmost relevance in this field due to preferences evidenced by older age groups and to insufficiencies exposed in most service platforms, such as lack of personalization and interaction features.

Keywords: Engagement platforms & engagement ecosystem ·
Ambient Assisted Living (AAL) · Ageing well · Digital and human advisors ·
Authorized Active Advisors · ICT

1 Introduction

The fast advances in the field of Information and Communication Technologies (ICT) have been inducing changes in the interactions among individuals within their environments. When taken from a consumer-company/consumer-organization inter-action's point of view, the various touch points have evolved over time and new technologies have acted as great enablers of service innovation [1]. ICT allows consumers to expect and receive more service, information and support than ever before. The experience of new platform technologies is significantly increasing consumers' expectations towards services and, more importantly, it is also promoting their empowerment. We are living in a new age of consumer engagement, which can be defined as the individual psychological state resulting from the interactions between a focal engagement subject – the consumer – and an object – the organization [2]. It has also been observed that consumers have demonstrated willingness to become more active and engaged in the value creation themselves [2]. Consequently, there is a demand for a transformation of this value creation in society in general, and in organizations providing products and/or services in particular.

An important market of service provision for the contemporary ageing society has opened for Ambient Assisted Living (AAL) solutions, targeting active and healthy ageing in the older adults' preferred environment. Those solutions take a significant slice of the so-called 'silver economy' [3], defined as "the sum of all economic activity serving the needs of those aged 50 and over including both the products and services they purchase directly and the further economic activity this spending generates" [3, p. 7]. This economy was foreseen to achieve 15 trillion dollars in 2020, globally [3]. In spite of its growing importance, it was previously noticed that services within this market are provided in isolation and often in a technocentric way [4]. These factors are likely to contribute, together with other factors, to the current gap between the technology development and its uptake by end users, particularly by the older age groups.

Considering the state of this problem, we begin by mentioning that organizations providing services in the AAL field must predominantly act as enablers of engagement platforms. Only in such capacities can they leverage individuals' and groups' drive to create value *for*, but mostly *with* them. For the implementation of those engagement platforms, the technological developments in the last 20 years have been instrumental by allowing interactions among stakeholders in virtual environments [5]. However, in the contemporary society, the consumer journey is growing in complexity in most service sectors, which requires increasingly sophisticated service logics [6]. Indeed, a number of ICT companies have been expanding their service portfolio from entirely virtual to additional physical experiences, a trend suggesting a certain shifting 'back' to the face-to-face (f2f) interaction, which opposes the purely virtual service landscapes. Notwithstanding the development of positive examples (e.g. Google and Microsoft business cases) a real, seamless merger of both physical and virtual worlds in the service user journey may still be some way off [5]. Hence, to discuss how to address those issues, we first elaborate on Breidbach and colleagues' [5] definition of 'engagement ecosystems', which considers both physical and virtual focal actor touch points, to argue that an integration of real/physical and virtual worlds is necessary for service provision in the AAL field. The challenge here is how to integrate both virtual and physical dimensions in an optimal solution for stakeholder engagement. For the consumer group of older adults, we need to take into consideration, firstly, the digital divide. This population group at present has no comprehensive access to the digital world. Services provided virtually only might prohibit their full participation. Secondly, this age group in particular shows a preference for f2f contact, usually perceived as more trustworthy [7, 8]. Thirdly, although often treated as a homogeneous group, older adults are actually a heterogeneous group with diverse needs and life contexts. In observing the ongoing debates, two further key points of concern emerge: *trust* and *personalization* in service provision. We argue that the integration of the two interaction interfaces (physical and virtual) and that functionalities, which support the collaboration between multiple stakeholders, facilitate trust building, and digitization can guarantee personalization to a certain extent.

This paper discusses the challenges of integrating the different interaction interfaces with respect to advisory services in the AAL field. Thereby, it reflects on results from the EU-funded ActiveAdvice project, which intends to set up a pan-European advisory and decision-support platform. This platform attempts to bring together available AAL products, services and stakeholders. By doing so, it seeks to evaluate how advice is going to be best provided. We further take into consideration a shift from a purely online interaction to an integrated logic, in the scope of advisory services targeted at stakeholders in the AAL ecosystem, towards the promotion of services and products which are, ideally, context and situation-aware, pro-active, and adaptive. In line with this, we will discuss the concept of human advisors, so-called 'Authorized Active Advisors', an idea born within the ActiveAdvice project and reinforced by the insights from user-centred requirement interviews conducted with multiple stakeholders [7, 8]. "I believe digital tools can enhance the advisor-investor relationship, not end it". [9] Here, the author stresses that technology is not going to replace the human advice, it will complement it. We start our discussions with a closer look at engagement ecosystems and engagement platforms; and we attempt to answer the questions of how an engagement ecosystem for AAL can integrate digital and human advice. This paper follows the previous publication of preliminary discussions in the paper "High Tech, High Touch: Integrating Digital and Human AAL Advisory Services for Older Adults" [10], which was presented at the ICT4AWE 2018 Conference.

2 Engagement Platforms Integrating Virtual and Real Environments

Ramaswamy and Gouillart [11] framed engagement platforms in the virtual sphere as purpose-built, ICT-enabled environments. Breidbach et al. [5] proposed an expansion of Ramaswamy's definition for engagement platforms by describing them as "physical or virtual focal actor touch points, which are designed to provide structural support for resource integration, and that intend to ensure co-creation in relation to a focal actor or object, in order to enhance an actors' [sic] ability to experience engagement with such focal object" [5, p. 7]. As exemplified by Blasco-Arcas et al. [12], engagement platforms can have a social focus, namely in online brand communities such as Harley-Davidson, or a socially driven approach to transactions as illustrated by Amazon's and Nike's social commerce platforms. Taking those definitions into account, the logical question is then to ask: What features must a platform have to be qualified as an engagement platform? Ramaswamy and Gouillart [11] characterize engagement platforms through (i) transparency (visible interactions for a wider audience); (ii) access (user opportunity to integrate resources); (iii) dialogue (exchange of information), and (iv) reflexivity (platform's adaptability to changes). Other published works tend to reproduce this view with a lack of scientific production being brought to attention.

2.1 Engagement Platforms in AAL Service Provision

Taking into account the features that a platform must have to qualify as an engagement platform, another question should be raised: If at all, to what extent are the current service platforms in the AAL field acting as engagement platforms? To kick-start the discussion on this question, we carried out a search and analysis of websites, portals and platforms that promote assistive technologies and services for older adults. Overall, the aim was to identify and analyse studies, concepts and best practices. First, the search was conducted on a selection of scientific databases (Jstor Emerald Insights, Web of Science, Science Direct, Taylor & Francis online) on the basis of defined keywords (e.g. AAL Services, Stakeholder AAL, AAL Feedback, Feedback Advisory, Trust Digital Advisory, Assistive Services, Social Features). In total, we screened 70 articles along the topics of (i) studies on AAL user information; (ii) platforms (discussed & evaluated in research/studies); (iii) user feedback and social features; (iv) digital support algorithms; and (v) authorization process [13]. Following this initial analysis, in a second phase, 42 articles were evaluated based on a thematic structure [14] with almost 600 codes assigned in order to categorise, cluster and organise common themes to compare [15, p. 318]. The selection of codes was clustered into the following main topics: structure and features, use and development of ICT (in healthcare), advice and feedback, care/healthcare, stakeholders, AAL (in general and in particular AAL platforms and service ecosystems). For each article, a short case description was added.

Second, a sample of twelve service platforms was selected to be analysed in detail regarding stakeholder involvement, interaction and feedback features: Aging Care (USA); National Association for Home Care & Hospice (USA); Parent giving (USA);

Make it ReAAL (Europe-Denmark, Germany, Italy, Netherlands, Norway, Spain); Silver Eco (France, Belgium), Pour les Personnes Âgées (France); Ooreka (France), Unforgettable (UK), AALIANCE 2 (Europe); Services Québec (Canada); and Independent Living Center (Australia). These were chosen because of their superordinate reach and influence. The authors are very well aware of various national solutions. The survey was not meant to be a complete and detailed account. The evaluation of the articles and later of the platforms was based on predetermined criteria: country of origin, stakeholders, type of service provided, promotion of ICT products, and accessibility of platform. We also looked into whether advice was provided to customers and, if so, how it was conducted (e.g. personalization features in advice provision).

Here, we present the key points that emerged regarding interaction and personalization for compelling engagement experiences. First, we conclude that less than one third of the articles analysed dealt explicitly with the development and establishment of platforms and online information portals. Also, none explicitly discussed a meta-AAL platform, which would be integrating services, products, and different stakeholders. This suggested that the establishment of platforms in the context of technology promotion for older adults is not a priority. From both the article analysis and the platform analysis, the existence of anything like an EU-wide AAL marketing platform was not identified. However, a positive aspect emerging from the analysis of the platforms under review revealed that the promotion of ICT and/or home care products and services as well as the sharing of information for older adults is of importance. Our key observations from the platform analysis are: first, clearly most of the platforms target older adults and their relatives, and thereby attempt to simply link manufacturers with potential consumers. Therefore, a multi-stakeholder perspective is generally missing. This is especially relevant in the context of AAL, as such an approach, leading to more collaboration and coordination among stakeholders, could help addressing the current challenges on solutions uptake by its primary end users [7, 8]. Second, among the twelve platforms, only eight guarantee immediate or direct feedback. They offer neither personalised feedback and/or advice nor interaction in the manner of e.g. a user forum. Third, user forums are widely missing; in these forums users would learn peer to peer about usage of devices, problems in using them and where to buy and ask for service. Fourth, if at all, price information is reduced to a price range only. Lastly, it must be stated that the platforms in focus were not comprehensively user-friendly. The minimum acceptable standard of age-friendly websites and platforms refers to simple interfaces and easy to feed and find content. Also, it must be stressed that platforms analysed are not clear about the user groups targeted by them.

2.2 Building Up Engagement Platforms

With respect to the building-up of an engagement platform, we argue that interactivity are the key elements on which to focus. Guaranteeing interactivity has, however, been proved challenging, especially when developing a platform that supports sharing of information, knowhow and products, as well as building up networks of different stakeholders. Yet, more and more people prefer to actively contribute rather than to only consume information from others in the online environment [12]. This was indeed one of the insights emerging from the requirement interviews carried out within the ActiveAdvice project, where consumers expressed interest in becoming more active users as well as commenters in online environments [7, 8]. This survey, with 38 semi-structured interviews, was carried out across six European Union member states with twelve consumers, fourteen businesses representatives and twelve government representatives [7, 8].

The more interactive platforms are, the more likely their users become providers of content "in the form of evaluations, recommendations, opinions, instructions, facts and experiences"[16, p. 467]. Correspondingly, the more interaction there is, the more users are willing to contribute to a platform [17]. Consequently, an engagement platform that has the potential to motivate users to actively generate content provides other users a richer and more up-to-date service. This kind of engagement has also proved to foster empowerment, as consumers become aware of their roles and influences [12]. Thus, the psychological attachment to an online community can be a strong driving force. Within a community, it is easier to ask for information, seek advice or obtain feedback [13]. From the consumers' perspective, these interactions are particularly relevant for empowering them through learning from other consumers' experiences and choices. Consumer-to-consumer (C2C) interaction facilitates the decision-making process, as it can help in diminishing the overload of information and the effort needed to filter it, therefore reducing uncertainty and complexity [18]. It seems that advice in form of contributions and reports by peers is a mean to generally increase trust in online advice. Hence, in this landscape, older adults and informal caregivers themselves have the opportunity to become 'advisors' on AAL solutions through experience sharing, thus upgrading their participation as content consumers to content generators. Indeed, from the user studies conducted for the ActiveAdvice project, we concluded that a common expectation from consumers is obtaining feedback about AAL solutions, preferably by other end users, offering personal experiences with products, services and the platform presenting the solutions [7, 8]. Information on the person presenting feedback is also an important aspect, for evaluating reliability, usefulness or trustworthiness [7, 8]. In addition, Bronner and Hoog [19] provide evidence that an active participation of consumers in the form of commenting can significantly influence the purchasing decisions of other users.

In our view, within the scope of an ICT-enabled environment, a platform must also provide multi-stakeholders' interaction, including mechanisms for consumer-to-organization (C2O) and C2C interaction. These provide stakeholders with the opportunity to participate, to create content and to connect, minimizing the drawbacks from lack of physical engagement in f2f service provision models and generating more "compelling engagement experiences" [20, p. 11, 21]. Interaction among stakeholders is, thus, a key to reduce the risk perceived in decision making and in general terms, to foster consumers' trust in an online environment.

The platform analysis (cf. Sect. 2.1) has shown that personalised feedback and advice is not yet common. However, we previously concluded that personalization is a key requirement [7, 8], and we understand that it is essential for building up an engagement platform. Firstly, it enables the recognition of the individual consumer's particular needs [22] and, if the online platform manages to provide personalization mechanisms, it secondly facilitates both the decision-making process and allows consumers to choose offers tailored to their needs. These are undoubtedly some of the requirements the ActiveAdvice project aims to fulfill, when proposing a pan-European advisory and support platform on AAL solutions. The AAL community will unprecedentedly benefit from a multi-stakeholder platform that also facilitates the interaction between different actors, the transfer of knowhow between them and an empowering of older adults.

3 Users in Need for Support: Challenges of Virtual and Real-Life Interaction

As online platforms annul the typical f2f interaction, the user's acceptance has to be a main concern and a high priority of developers and promoters. However, it is a well-known problem that what is possible from a technological point of view and what is assumed from the developer side must not necessarily meet the individual user's needs. "(F)for a service to be successful it must be provided under consideration of these criteria: the right good (product or service), in the right quantity and quality, at the right time, and the right place for the right customer at the right price" [23, p. 78]. Furthermore, there are quite high expectations towards the services provided through online platforms. We also need to take into consideration that the use of the internet is often reduced to a first consultancy rather than for ongoing advice. Yet, especially questions about health issues, which are considered as private, are a reason for preferred online consultancy in relative anonymity. Concerning older adults, research has shown that the fear of losing interpersonal contacts, thus aggravating loneliness, can be connected to a minor adhesion to online platforms, if those are connected to purely virtual service provision [7, 8, 24–27]. However, it has been reported that if technologies are seen as facilitators of new social interactions rather than replacing mechanisms of human interactions, this fear of losing social contacts can be minimized [28].

Based on a comprehensive, user-centred view of the constraints and facilitators for interactions in the virtual world within a decision-support platform, we argue that older adults can benefit from the integration of digital and human advice on AAL solutions, as a system that can capitalize the benefits and strengths of both advice formats. Studies have supported, for example, the strong impact of virtual agents in the context of online-shopping, in addressing age related navigational needs [29]. Similar results are known from medical research. Rather than the idea of virtual agents, the need to navigate users towards useful online information is discussed. This can be done by physicians and other healthcare experts [30].

Moreover, within the context of the ActiveAdvice project, business representatives stressed the 'neutral' nature of digital advice mechanisms when it comes to guiding a consumer towards the solution fitting his/her needs [7, 8]. Despite the benefits of digital advice, there are some distinct challenges that need to be overcome. First, from a digital-human advisory integration point of view, an already stressed pragmatic argument relies on the fact that the digital divide still is a well-known challenge affecting older age groups, albeit in an unbalanced way across European countries. Contributing factors are poor ICT skills, fear of both the technology itself and the learning process, and a lack of financial resources to purchase devices and internet access [28, 31–34].

Furthermore, there are barriers preventing older adults from accessing and engaging with ICT environments. These barriers still concern the older adults' and caregivers' lack of ICT knowledge and skills, and their sometimes limited or restricted access to the internet and/or to a web-enabled device. Additionally, negative attitudes towards technology, difficulties measuring risks online and the reluctance to purchase online can prevent older adults from engaging in the digital world. Other barriers as well as perceived risks are associated with the design of online platforms themselves, the quality of the information provided, the presence/absence of rating systems and with the lack of trust in services provided online (e.g. fear of manipulation, fraud and extortion). Negative assumptions are also single design elements that distract or overwhelm users [35]. If these kinds of barriers are well documented, it is also accepted that, to a certain extent, they will tend to decrease in future generations, especially with regards to lack of ICT skills [36]. Investigating the two age cohorts, the digital natives (the Millennials), and the digital immigrants (the Baby Boomers), Bart et al. [in 37, p. 47] concluded that age is a critical dimension when it comes to trust on online interactions. Millennials value time saving, e.g. navigation enabling a quick search of information, easy findings and shorter response times. Baby Boomers prefer security of their personal data. While Millennials appreciate information about the product and the seller right on the site, Baby Boomers do not trust the sellers' promotional materials and are more likely to look for consumer feedback. Millennials in particular are used to participate in virtual communities and in seeking consultancy with virtual experts [in 37, p. 47].

Yet, as the focus of AAL is on very specific needs of a specific user group, an AAL platform always will have to assure the integration of the virtual and real life. However, even if it is demonstrated that e-services for older adults need to take the potential impact of generational differences on online trust into consideration, we argue that the ICT uptake actually depends on the intersection of multiple factors. These are related with both technology features and users' characteristics (e.g. age, gender, physical or cognitive skills, expectations, biographical experience) [38].

A second challenge to overcome is the fact that besides idiosyncrasies regarding older adults' preferences towards both digital and physical worlds, growing old and being in need of support is usually rather a local or regional experience, even if projects are generally carried out in an international atmosphere. Thus, an interactive, highly flexible, approved and continuously updated platform needs to take the above mentioned aspects into consideration. The platform should be able to support people with very specific needs in their regional contexts, as well as giving them access to an international community and knowledge base. Such complex logic in an optimal service provision to older adults is probably only achievable by using the 'human touch'. In fact, requirement interviews for the ActiveAdvice project have shown that in spite of the stakeholders' recognition of the high value of an online advisory platform, both consumers and business representatives stated that getting advice online still competes with the f2f experience. For customers, it is perceived as more trustworthy, while for companies it is seen as bedrock for consumers to engage and build a relationship with the company [7, 8].

A third argument summarizes what was stated earlier: An integration of real and virtual environments in engagement ecosystems enables C2C interactions. The co-creation of value is thus facilitated [5]. This, our fourth argument, enhances user trust on the services provided, both advice services or any others. Trust is certainly one of the most critical user/consumer issues [17], and one of the motives for supporting investments in digital-physical integration for service provision. In the digital sphere, consumers need to trust the website, the communication by this mean and finally, if products are promoted on the website, in the products themselves. In AAL, trust was shown as a key attitudinal factor for solutions' uptake [26]. From the requirement interviews carried out within the ActiveAdvice project, we drew similar conclusions and found that trust is, according to the stakeholders' point of view, influenced by: the communication strategy and the web-layout; the perception of neutrality regarding the information provided and the individuals providing that information; the perceived quality of that information; the access to real users' feedback; and the perception that feedbacks are 'fair', i.e. not exclusively guided by negative incentives [7, 8]. Without a doubt, the presence of e.g. provider advice, privacy cues and community features have a high influence on trust in online platforms [37, p. 48]. Overall, we need to take into consideration that one obstacle for acquiring health information online by older adults is the perception that information available online has low quality, can be biased or misleading, is frequently unprofessionally run, omits peer-reviewed materials by independent actors, and the selection of the most reliable and suitable information is constrained by information overload on health issues [33]. Moreover, data security and data privacy, ethical and cultural issues as well as market development and legal regulations are crucial aspects that need to be considered to stir up trust. In summary, users are confronted with many complexities while using online advisory services, which they hardly know how to manage. Therefore, knowing how to build-up trust and identifying the drivers of online trust are key responsibilities in service provision.

4   Integration of Human and Digital Advice – The ActiveAdvice Approach

The arguments exposed above strongly indicate that a platform, which aims to provide decision-support on AAL products and services, and as a matter of fact any platform for AAL products and services, cannot be a stand-alone solution. Rather, it has to be part of an integrated and systematic service logic, incorporating both virtual and physical service formats, which promote the integration of different actors with different interests and contributions. As previously outlined: "People – whether consumers or service providers – are complex agents, with highly diverse cognitive frameworks, values and attitudes, physical and emotional needs (…) Service systems are therefore complex to model and manage – but they may also be resilient and innovative. People can be empowered to act in non-mechanical ways, responding to unexpected circumstances and collaborating to solve problems. They can be linked together in new ways through new information technology" [39, p. 417]. In the scope of advisory services on AAL solutions, we argue for the integration of digital and human advice. A lesson learned from the financial sector, where robo-advisers help people with their investments, is that they are not really advisors. This is because they lack emotions: "While AI software programs can analyze vast amounts of information, recognize sophisticated patterns, learn and automatically update their models, they leave investors unassisted or without emotional help." [40, p. 255]. In short, people sometimes just want to talk, want to learn from other people's experiences, need to have explanations embedded in broader contexts. That is true for the finance industry as well as for every other context where people are in need for support.

In fact, within the ActiveAdvice project, we conceptualized the human advisor as an assistant for users helping in informed decision-making – a human addition to the digital advisory logic in the ICT platform. These so-called 'Authorized Active Advisors' are then foreseen to assist individuals in finding the right solution for their problem or needs, complementing the digital platform. Using the ActiveAdvice platform, which provides the 'Authorized Active Advisors' with the necessary information, they will create a distinct added value to the digital platform, such as: (i) contributing to awareness raising on AAL in general; (ii) bridging the knowledge gap, especially with context-adapted knowledge, i.e. knowledge adapted to the local settings; (iii) providing personal contact, addressing older adults' preferences and promoting trust; (iv) filling possible gaps in the digital advisor system; (v) providing a more in-depth, individual and personalised decision support; (vi) populating the platform with professional feedback/testimony and follow-up on satisfaction with products or solutions; and (vii) stimulate and support users to provide feedback on the platform.

In order to allow them to provide the necessary advisory services, the human advisor workflow follows a five-step procedure, as also illustrated in the figure below (cf. Fig. 1): (i) 'Authorized Active Advisors' listen to the need and translate it into a search strategy that complements the digital advisory component; (ii) they identify solutions and suppliers and assess their pertinence; (iii) they assist the individual in making the decision; (iv) they follow-up on satisfaction and stimulate users to provide a feedback on the platform; and (v) they feed the platform with professional feedback or testimonies [41].

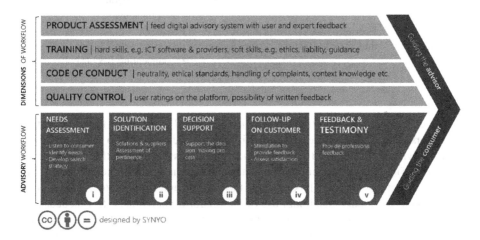

Fig. 1. Human advisor workflow following a five-step procedure.

This human advisor workflow was conceived as being based on the following four dimensions as included in Fig. 1 (cf. Table 1):

Table 1. Dimensions of the human advisor workflow.

Assessment of products and services	AAL products and services are all the time updated and assessed – based on the digital advice fed by user and expert feedback.	
Training	• Make advisors familiar with the platform and the TAALXONOMY [see 42]; • Provide target group-specific training (according to the different needs); • Focus on the decision-making process and how to enhance the quality of decisions; • Offer guidance with respect to the creation of a human network around the digital community of the platform	**Training Curricula** (covering a skills set and basic knowledge): *Hard skills* • Theory on ageing, active and healthy ageing; • ICT basics; • Overview of AAL products and services (applications, main features and technical issues); • ActiveAdvice platform usage to provide the best advice; • AAL products and services budgeting *Soft skills* • Advising skills, • Ethics and liabilities
Code of Conduct	Applying a co-designed code of conduct as a mean to control and manage the quality of the interaction between offer (providers) and demand (users, consumers)	**Requirements** • Neutrality • Compliance with minimum ethical standards • Acceptance to follow the code of conduct • Complete recording and handling of complaints
Quality Control (products & services)	User feedback on the platform directly (quantitative and qualitative)	**Feedback** • Scoring • Commenting [see 41]

The code of conduct and training are the two central elements of the accreditation of advisors. The ActiveAdvice platform will also provide services to the 'Authorized Active Advisors', including (i) maintenance and access to the platform and all its resources; (ii) regular information on updates and on innovations entering the market (on the platform or through linking with the AAL market observatory); (iii) initial training on how to make maximum use of the platform via partners; (iv) feedback on satisfaction and experience with solutions, products and service as well as suppliers; and (v) handling of complaints. However, the most crucial issue within the concept, even when the Authorized Active Advisors' role and workflows are globally well defined, is to clarify who actually should provide advice to consumers. Within the

ActiveAdvice project, we identified four possible profiles: (i) professionals in the process of assisting older people (e.g. occupational therapists, care workers, architects); (ii) volunteers (including retired persons interested in AAL solutions and associates of user associations); (iii) public sector employees (e.g. within a municipality, or other sectors such as home adaption, energy etc.); and (iv) suppliers of solutions. In the ongoing process of the project, the last profile – suppliers of solutions – was challenged.

As a result from our requirements analysis for the ActiveAdvice project [7, 8], we were able to define characteristics of the Authorized Active Advisors profile. There is a need for neutrality of the Authorized Active Advisor; this is a shared concern by all targeted groups – older adults and their caregivers, business and government representatives. However, for business actors, a paradoxical position emerged: while advice is perceived as being best given by those who sell a product, it can lead to disruptions in the neutrality condition. A solution to this problem could be the establishment of older adult panels to test products and services as well as the platform itself. Similarly, volunteers could act as advisors on the platform. Authorized Active Advisors must be able to promote stakeholder involvement, interactivity and trust. And they must be capable of translating needs into a search strategy, of identifying solutions, of providing decision support and follow-ups as well as feedback after the purchase. For each profile, e.g. for an architect giving advice to volunteers offering their help, an understanding of roles, responsibilities and communication logics need to be further established.

Based on a preliminary research we can provide a first answer to the questions: (i) who are the human advisors; (ii) what kind of knowledge do they need, to become Authorized Active Advisors; and (iii) what kind of training is necessary to provide this knowledge? A set of semi-structured interviews (n = 5) was carried out with employees of the municipality of Alkmaar (the Netherlands). The interview analysis shows that there is a preference for a human advisor profile with a background in care provision, or that human advisors are employees of organisations supporting older adults. Furthermore, they should have (or be trained to gain) basic knowledge of healthcare and healthcare technologies as well as training on technologies for ageing independently in general. Most importantly, 'Authorized Active Advisors' have to be able to identify the specific problems or challenges related to certain health issues, and in line with this, the relations between specific diseases and possible technological devices that might solve or reduce these health problems. One core value any human advisor need to provide is, again, trust, as well as the integration of a multi-stakeholder perspective, which at the same time are considered main challenges. Naturally, the human advisor approach will also support the personalisation of the decision-support, which is a third core value. Furthermore, the human advisors allow extending the interactivity of the platform and improving or facilitating the aspect of 'dialogue', i.e. the exchange of information, which is one of the core elements outlined by Ramaswamy and Gouillart [11]. Still, because of the complexity and the many open questions related to human advice and its importance for older adults, and due to the fact that different advisor profiles are probable to emerge in different local realities, further research is necessary.

5 Conclusions

The platform analysis first discussed in this article suggested that current service platforms promoting AAL technologies and services for older adults lack in most parts to provide either personalization and/or interaction opportunities among stakeholders, including C2O and C2C interaction. We consider these interaction mechanisms to be strong requirements for promoting 'true' engagement platforms. In the AAL field, engagement platforms not only have the potential to promote AAL products and services but also to empower and engage stakeholders, as well as to facilitate the co-creation of value. Also, by considering the complexity in service logics nowadays, we argue that an engagement ecosystem for AAL, especially regarding advisory services for AAL solutions, must integrate both digital and human advice. In this context, the shift from a purely online to an integrated service logic is a path to enhance stakeholders' trust in advisory services. We also argue that following this approach, older adults will be provided with those AAL products and services that are best suited to the individual and local/national context.

With a focus on the 'human touch', we conceptualized the 'Authorized Active Advisors' as human agents providing assistance to users of the ActiveAdvice platform. We argue that those actors are of utmost importance due to, first, the preferences previously revealed by older adults: those actors can answer to stakeholders' preferences for f2f contact, substantiated by the human interaction role in establishing trusty consumer-organization relationships. Second, the 'Authorized Active Advisors' have the potential to mitigate the insufficiencies detected in current service platforms, e.g. the lack of personalized information and feedback. Furthermore, the 'Authorized Active Advisors' might also hold great importance in the creation of an engagement ecosystem, where synergies between primary end users, providers, governmental agencies and other types of stakeholders can be established and sustained. In an AAL ecosystem, trained and independent human advisors are required to safeguard trust in advisory services and, consequently, favour the adhesion to those services. We already can stress the need for crucial soft and hard skills to be promoted as an 'Authorized Active Advisors' candidate. A refinement of the 'Authorized Active Advisors' skill profile is foreseen for the near future, fed by consultancy with multiple stakeholders. In a next step, training curricula will be established, to be piloted with interested parties.

Another important issue to bear in mind regarding the 'Authorized Active Advisor' figure is: Are human advisors also capable of reducing the potential aversion and rejection of technology? The latter is often linked to the lower experience with technology older adults might have, but also with the idea of technology substituting human interaction in service provision. In linking technology promoted via an online platform with human advisory, we, in a way, oppose the frequently associated isolation and loneliness fear of older adults. Human advisors can help to overcome these fears, can encourage older adults to participate in digital communities, also with the intent of minimizing the digital divide, which is still affecting this age-group. In order to be an adequate complement to digital advice, those human advisors will always have to consider the heterogeneous profiles of older adults and the unique features of each local context.

It is vital for the successful implementation of the ActiveAdvice platform and the advisory service that further research will take place to better understand the usage of different channels in the advisory of AAL solutions – from direct f2f interaction to phone support or to online interaction via chats or forums. Therefore, this and the earlier mentioned questions – who should be the human advisors, what kind of knowledge and training should those advisors have? – will be more thoroughly investigated in a next step within the ActiveAdvice project. We aim to challenge the initial results obtained in a set of interviews carried in the Municipality of Alkmaar (cf. Sect. 4). In this sense, workshops and additional interviews are planned to happen in the near future, in all participating countries (Austria, the Netherlands, Belgium, Portugal, Great Britain and Switzerland). These data collection moments will be carried out with care professionals, architects, and individuals from all age groups who can act as volunteers to assist their peers in living longer at home; public administration; suppliers of solutions, including retailers (e.g. alarm systems, hearing aid) who might become 'Authorized Active Advisors' as an advanced service for their customers; and other relevant stakeholders previously mapped for each partner country. The ActiveAdvice solution is expected to offer a subscription area where human advisors can sign in to have access to all the functionalities an information hosted in the ActiveAdvice platform (not just the basic functionalities offered). Finally, it is crucial to understand what and to what extend local or regional knowledge, which is, as outlined above, crucial for the nature of ageing and hold also implications regarding access to AAL solutions (e.g. local funding schemes), must be provided.

Overall, when it comes to the development of an integrated system for advisory services on AAL, we recommend the promotion of engagement ecosystems where multiple stakeholders' profiles evolve together. Moreover, we favour a symbiotic approach combining human and digital advisory, which allows personalised guidance and reduced complexity in search operations and decision support. Feedback and evaluation mechanisms are a 'must-have' in order to create social awareness and a sense of community regarding C2O and C2C interactions. The potentials of human advice for online engagement platforms on AAL products and services are, indeed, to be explored. We contribute, with the present and future research and development work, to bridge this gap while taking into account different national, if not to say, regional specifics. The ActiveAdvice platform is on its way. In combining human and digital advisory services, the platform service is able to truly build up on the best of both worlds, complementing the weaknesses and building on the strengths of both digital and human AAL advisory services for older adults.

Acknowledgements. The authors would like to acknowledge the co-financing by the European Commission AAL Joint Programme and the related national agencies in Austria, Belgium, the Netherlands, Portugal, Switzerland and the United Kingdom. One of the authors (Soraia Teles) is also individually supported by the Portuguese Foundation for Science And Technology (FCT; D/BD/135496/2018; Phd Program in Clinical and Health Services Research (PDICSS).

References

1. Breidbach, C.F., Maglio, P.P.: A service science perspective on the role of ICT in service innovation. In: ECIS (2015)
2. Brodie, R.J., Hollebeek, L.D., Jurić, B., Ilić, A.: Customer engagement: conceptual domain, fundamental propositions and implications for research. J. Serv. Res. **14**(3), 252–271 (2011)
3. European Commission: Growing the European Silver Economy (2015). http://ec.europa.eu/research/innovation-union/pdf/active-healthy-ageing/silvereco.pdf
4. Baldissera, T.A., Camarinha-Matos, L.M.: Towards a collaborative business ecosystem for elderly care. In: Camarinha-Matos, L.M., Falcão, A.J., Vafaei, N., Najdi, S. (eds.) DoCEIS 2016. IAICT, vol. 470, pp. 24–34. Springer, Cham (2016). https://doi.org/10.1007/978-3-319-31165-4_3
5. Breidbach, C.F., Brodie, R., Hollebeek, L.: Beyond virtuality: from engagement platforms to engagement ecosystems. Manag. Serv. Qual. 24(6), 592–611 (2014)
6. Peters, Ch., Blohm, I., Leimeister, J.M.: Anatomy of successful business models for complex services: insights from the telemedicine field. J. Manag. Inf. Syst. **32**(3), 75–104 (2015)
7. Teles, S., Bertel, D., Kofler, A.Ch., Ruscher, S.H., Paúl, C.: A Multi-perspective view on AAL stakeholders' needs. a user-centred requirement analysis for the ActiveAdvice european project. In: 2017 International Conference on Information and Communication Technologies for Ageing Well and e-Health (ICT4AWE) (2017)
8. Teles, S., Kofler, Andrea Ch., Schmitter, P., Ruscher, S., Paúl, C., Bertel, D.: ActiveAdvice: a multi-stakeholder perspective to understand functional requirements of an online advice platform for AAL products and services. In: Röcker, C., O'Donoghue, J., Ziefle, M., Maciaszek, L., Molloy, W. (eds.) ICT4AWE 2017. CCIS, vol. 869, pp. 168–190. Springer, Cham (2018). https://doi.org/10.1007/978-3-319-93644-4_9
9. Roy, S.: Will technology eventually replace human financial advisors? (2016). https://www.blog.invesco.us.com/will-robo-advisor-replace-human-financial-advisors/
10. Bertel, D., et al.: High tech, high touch: integrating digital and human AAL advisory services for older adults. In: Proceedings of the 4th International Conference on Information and Communication Technologies for Ageing Well and e-Health - Volume 1: ICT4AWE, pp. 241–249 (2018). ISBN 978-989-758-299-8. https://doi.org/10.5220/0006799002410249
11. Ramaswamy, V., Gouillart, F.: Building the co-creative enterprise. Harv. Bus. Rev. **88**(10), 100–109 (2010)
12. Blasco-Arcas, L., Blasco-Arcas, L., Hernandez-Ortega, B.I., Hernandez-Ortega, B.I., Jimenez-Martinez, J., Jimenez-Martinez, J.: Engagement platforms: the role of emotions in fostering customer engagement and brand image in interactive media. J. Serv. Theory Pract. **26**(5), 559–589 (2016)
13. Kofler, A.Ch., Awuku-Sao, G., Schmitter, P.: Baseline report on AAL advice, decision and authorization. D2.1, ActiveAdvice AAL Programme Project No. 851908 (2016)
14. Nadin, S., Cassell, C.: Using data matrices. In: Cassell, C., Symon, G.G. (eds.) Essential Guide to Qualitative Methods in Organizational Research, pp. 271–287. Sage, Thousand Oaks (2004)
15. Flick, U.: An Introduction to Qualitative Research. Sage, Thousand Oaks (2009)
16. Sheng, X., Zolfagharian, M.: Consumer participation in online product recommendation services: augmenting the technology acceptance model. J. Serv. Mark. **28**(6), 460–470 (2014)
17. Cummins, Sh., Peltier, J., Schibrowsky, J., Nill, A.: Consumer behavior in the online context. J. Res. Interact. Mark. **8**(3), 169–202 (2014)

18. Miceli, G., Ricotta, F., Costabile, M.: Customizing customization: a conceptual framework for interactive personalization. J. Interact. Mark. **21**(2), 6–25 (2007)
19. Bronner, F.A., de Hoog, R.: Consumer-generated versus marketer-generated websites in consumer. Int. J. Mark. Res. **52**(2), 231–248 (2010)
20. Ramaswamy, V.: Co-creation of value: towards an expanded paradigm of value creation. Mark. Rev. St Gall. **26**(6), 11–17 (2009)
21. Montgomery, A.L., Smith, M.D.: Prospects for personalization on the internet. J. Interact. Mark. **23**(2), 130–137 (2009)
22. Füller, J., Matzler, K.: Virtual product experience and customer participation – a chance for customer-centred, really new products. Technovation **27**(6–7), 378–387 (2007)
23. Kriegel, J., Schmitt-Rüth, S., Güntert, B., Mallory, P.: New service development in German and Austrian health care – bringing e-health services into the market. Int. J. Healthc. Manag. **6**(2), 77–86 (2013). https://doi.org/10.1179/2047971913y.0000000034
24. Damodaran, L., Olphert, W.: User responses to assisted living technologies (ALTs) – a review of the literature. J. Integr. Care **18**(2), 25–32 (2010). https://doi.org/10.5042/jic.2010.0133
25. Novitzky, P., et al.: A review of contemporary work on the ethics of ambient assisted living technologies for people with dementia. Sci. Eng. Ethics **21**(3), 707–765 (2015). https://doi.org/10.1007/s11948-014-9552-x
26. Olphert, W., Damodaran, L., Balatsoukas, P., Parkinson, C.: Process requirements for building sustainable digital assistive technology for older people. J. Assist. Technol. **3**(3), 4–13 (2009)
27. Siegel, C., Hochgatterer, A., Dorner, T.E.: Contributions of ambient assisted living for health and quality of life in the elderly and care services – a qualitative analysis from the experts' perspective of care service professionals. BMC Geriatr. **14**(1) (2014). https://doi.org/10.1186/1471-2318-14-112
28. Lewin, D., et al.: Assisted living technologies for older and disabled people in 2030. Annexes to a draft final report to Ofcom. Plum Consulting, London (2010). https://www.ofcom.org.uk/__data/assets/pdf_file/0033/44889/assistedannexes.pdf
29. Rickel, J., Johnson, W.L.: Task-oriented collaboration with embodied agents in virtual worlds. In: Cassell, J., Cassell, J., Sullivan, J., Prevost, S., Churchill, E.F. (eds.) Embodied Conversational Agents, pp. 95–122. MIT Press, Boston (2000)
30. Lee, K., Hoti, K., Hughes, J.D., Emmerton, L.: Dr Google and the consumer: a qualitative study exploring the navigational needs and online health information-seeking behaviors of consumers with chronic health conditions. J. Med. Internet Res. **16**(12), e262 (2014). https://doi.org/10.2196/jmir.3706
31. Doyle, J., Bailey, C., Ni Scanaill, C., van den Berg, F.: Lessons learned in deploying independent living technologies to older adults' homes. Univers. Access Inf. Soc. (2013). https://doi.org/10.1007/s10209-013-0308-1
32. Finn, R.L., Wright, D.: Mechanisms for stakeholder coordination in ICT and ageing. J. Inf. Commun. Ethics Soc. **9**(4), 265–286 (2011). https://doi.org/10.1108/14779961111191066
33. Marschollek, M., Mix, S., Wolf, K.-H., Effertz, B., Haux, R., Steinhagen-Thiessen, E.: ICT-based health information services for elderly people: past experiences, current trends, and future strategies. Med. Inform. Internet Med. **32**(4), 251–261 (2007). https://doi.org/10.1080/14639230701692736
34. Sanders, C., et al.: Exploring barriers to participation and adoption of telehealth and telecare within the whole system demonstrator trial: a qualitative study. BMC Health Serv. Res. **12**(1) (2012). https://doi.org/10.1186/1472-6963-12-220
35. Kofler, A.Ch., Schmitter, P.: User requirements, decision workflow and use cases report. D2.3, ActiveAdvice AAL Programme Project No. 851908 (2017)

36. Reginatto, B.M.B.: Understanding barriers to wider telehealth adoption in the home environment of older people: an exploratory study in the Irish context. J. Adv. Life Sci. **4** (3,4), 63–76 (2012)
37. Obal, M., Kunz, W.: Trust development in e-services: a cohort analysis of Millennials and Baby Boomers. J. Serv. Manag. **24**(1), 45–63 (2013)
38. Nedopil, C., Schauber, C., Glende I.: AAL stakeholders and their requirement. Report by the Ambient and Assisted Living Association (2013)
39. Cardoso, C., et al.: Platform to support the development of information services for in-formal and formal care. In: Proceedings of the International Conference on Health Informatics, pp. 417–421 (2014)
40. Beltramini, E.: Human vulnerability and robo-advisory: An application of Coeckelbergh's vulnerability to the machine-human interface. Balt. J. Manag. **13**(2), 250–263 (2018). https://doi.org/10.1108/BJM-10-2017-0315
41. Denis, A.: Human Advisor Workflow. D3.4, ActiveAdvice AAL Programme Project No. 851908 (2017)
42. Leitner, P., et al.: TAALXONOMY. Entwicklung einer praktikablen Taxonomie zur effektiven Klassifizierung von AAL-Produkten und Dienstleitungen. Studienbericht (2015)

"In Clarity We Trust!" - An Empirical Study of Factors that Affect the Credibility of Health-Related Information on Websites

Luisa Vervier[✉], André Calero Valdez, and Martina Ziefle

Human Computer Interaction Center, RWTH Aachen University,
Campus Boulevard 57, Aachen, Germany
{vervier,calero-valdez,ziefle}@comm.rwth-aachen.de
http://www.comm.rwth-aachen.de/

Abstract. *"In case of side effects please consult your physician or pharmacist",* used to be the advice for questions regarding the intake of medicine or other health-related issues. Nowadays, the Internet has become the favored place to find this kind of information. However, the quality of online health information is mixed. This becomes an issue when people use online information for important health decisions. According to which criteria do users select the found information? To understand which elements on a website convince people to trust the information or not, we have conducted a study with two objectives: first, to identify factors that trigger credibility; second, to investigate to what extent both the media presentation and the severity of the associated disease influence the assessment of credibility. Possible factors were first collected in three focus groups (N = 17) and then operationalized in a questionnaire. We collected 184 responses, presenting and evaluating three different health websites with different disease complexity and severity (mild vs. life-threatening). The results show that complex information is preferred for more serious diseases. In addition, the disease has a significant influence on the criteria.

Keywords: Digital health information · Credibility factors · User-diversity · Ehealth · Health literacy

1 Introduction

In times of digitization, the Internet plays a dominant role in people's lives. In addition to the use for communication and entertainment reasons, the Internet is a medium for information search. The development of digital information is increasing. Day by day, the available information increases in quantity. Information about e.g., places, people, hours, or news are just a few search topics. One of the most sought areas is health issues [1]. Above all, due to a new awareness of health and lifestyle (i.e., quantified self) and the development of informed

© Springer Nature Switzerland AG 2019
P. D. Bamidis et al. (Eds.): ICT4AWE 2018, CCIS 982, pp. 83–107, 2019.
https://doi.org/10.1007/978-3-030-15736-4_5

patients, information is more relevant than ever. In addition to being informed only about health issues, people also take information as the basis for decisions about treatment or the intake of medicines [2]. Digital health information offers many benefits. Health information is always and available everywhere. It gives many people access to medical information [3]. People can actively participate in health issues and even collaborate with other people who are working on the same topic [4]. However, disadvantages of so much information circulating on the Internet are also present. Much of the information found online is non-serious or outright false and not recognized as being false or outdated [3]. Therefore, there may be psychological or physical consequences that may be incurred by relying on e.g., medical advice or false intake of medicine [5]. Therefore, it is a major challenge for health information researchers to evaluate the quality and credibility of websites [6]. People focus on different criteria for assessing information as correct [7]. There is a growing need to understand how this information is accessed and how it is used. What criteria are important for people's decision to trust the information? On the other hand, how diverse are the users? Which user prefers what kind of presentation? In this study we examine this kind of question. The aim of the study is to find out and to understand to what extent the media representation of health websites and the degree of the described disease play a role in their assessment. The study also aims to understand what kind of user characteristics affect the site's rating. This article—which extends upon earlier work [8]—is structured as follows: After this introduction, the current state of health information on the Internet, quality of health-related websites, credibility factors of health-related information, e-health literacy, and privacy concerns considering general search behavior are presented. Section 3 describes the research questions that guide the study as well as the research methodology. Section 4 presents the focus group approach regarding the generation of credibility factors, whereas Sect. 5 describes the questionnaire approach with respect to the research questions. Section 6 discusses the results and guidelines for website developers. Section 6.1 concludes this article with a brief discussion of the limitations of this work and an outlook on other research questions.

2   Related Work

In order to answer the questions that we address, we must first understand the state of the art in digital health information (see Sect. 2.1). Further, it is necessary to understand how quality of health related websites can be described (see Sect. 2.2). And since users perceive these quality aspects differently and turn them into credibility factors for health-related information (see Sect. 2.3) understanding what drives these differences is crucial. One core skill that determines the quality of this process is the concept of e-health literacy (see Sect. 2.4). Additionally, users have different privacy concerns and needs for privacy, which also impact search behavior (see Sect. 2.5). The following sections aim to provide an overview of how these topics interrelate to each other to motivate our research questions.

2.1 Digital Health Information

Information about health is often searched for online. More than 70% of people search the Internet for such information [1]. Most people conduct searches about their own health problems. Key topics include disease symptoms, prognoses, and treatment options [9]. In a study by Kienhus et al. [10] 61% of users who examined the impact of online patient search on patient-physiological interaction reported that the information they sought affected their own health. This finding underscores the need to understand people's reasons for evaluating information as trustworthy whenever it affects their health.

2.2 Quality of Health-Related Websites

Health information is often accessed on the Internet. Although many tools and policies already exist to obtain high-quality information [11], health-related information and its quality still fluctuate widely across the Internet [12]. Aspects of lack of information quality reveal a wide range of information that is not serious, out-of-date, or contain incorrect information. In addition, websites often serve as a platform for advertising rather than a platform for evidence-based sources. One of the biggest challenges for information seekers is therefore to evaluate the present information. But not only the content, but also the presentation of information such as layout, structure, images, etc. are aspects that influence the evaluation by the user.

2.3 Credibility Factors of Health-Related Information

The overdose of information that appears online when looking for information about health issues on the Internet is overwhelming. However, people have developed their own search behavior and when it comes to, e.g., health information sites, people focus on specific aspects. Which so-called credibility factors make digital information useful and trustworthy? Many studies have been conducted regarding this phenomenon. Eysenbach and Köhler [13] report that, for example, references, information on the latest update, as well as information on authors and images become important credibility factors of credible websites. In addition, information on alternative treatment options and side effects on health-related websites are additional credibility factors [14]. Benigeri and Pluye [15] have developed an approach to describe support criteria for the quality assessment of health-related digital information. Although there are already numerous catalogs of credibility factors, the quality rating still varies. It seems that user diversity strongly determines the importance of various aspects. Barnes et al. [16] found that, e.g., the extent of personal involvement has an impact on the evaluation of information. Less involved people seem to focus more on layout than content and timeliness, as is the case with more health-related stakeholders. In addition, younger people focus more on website layout [17] than older people who are more interested in references [18]. Our study aims to review these results and to identify more specific aspects taking into account user diversity.

2.4 eHealth Literacy

In addition to objective criteria such as the above-mentioned credibility factors, subjective ability factors play an important role in the evaluation of digital health information. Literacy is a very important aspect. People who are able to read and write have higher education, integrate and participate more easily in social life, and are able to understand and execute a greater degree of control over everyday events [19]. The term "eHealth literacy" describes the ability to search, find, read, understand, and evaluate health information from electronic sources. It means that people have the ability to apply the knowledge they have acquired and to address or solve a health problem [20]. Greater health literacy correlates with better health outcomes. Health literacy influences the use of health care, patient-physician relationship, and self-care [21]. It is obvious that the evaluation of digital health information differs strongly due to the individual differences in competence. To find out about the phenomenon of health literacy, it is integrated into our study.

2.5 Online Privacy

Hand in hand with the search for health-related online information goes the growing concern of the users' online information privacy. Whereas the online search for health-related topics allows user to ask sensitive or detailed question without the risk of facing judgment or stigma [22], in the same time people start worrying about their personal information which they leave behind when looking for some specific health issues. As personal information becomes more accessible, users worry that institutions and especially insurance companies misuse the information that is collected while users are online [23]. However, the level of awareness varies just as much as different users are. To find out to what extent users looking for online information also give additional thought to their privacy, we considered to include the phenomena of privacy concern and need for privacy in our study.

3   Question Addressed and Logic of Empirical Procedure

This paper raises the question of how digital health information is judged by its recipient and how it varies with the severity of the disease. In particular, the focus is on the perceived credibility of various media representations of websites, which are also influenced by two different degrees of severity of the disease. The purpose of the paper is to identify credibility factors that affect the recipient's attitude of trusting a health information website. Guidelines for site developers are presented based on the results. In order to identify, evaluate and quantify these factors, a two-way multi-method approach was chosen. In a first step, the data was collected qualitatively according to focus groups. Three focus groups were run with three different age groups. Since the methodical approach of the focus groups intended to collect different opinions of people's point of view, very general questions were guiding the group discussion:

1. *Where do you look for health-related information?*
2. *Which factors make information appear credible?*

Based on the results, a questionnaire was developed and the data was collected quantitatively. Questions guiding the questionnaire approach were:

1. *What are the key trust elements of a website that presents health information in general? Do age and gender influence the evaluation of credibility factors? Are the credibility factors different in relation to the severity of the disease?*
2. *To what extent does the media representation of a health website and the degree of the disease play a role in the opinion of the user?*
3. *To what extent do user factors such as age and gender influence the assessment of health information of varying severity?*

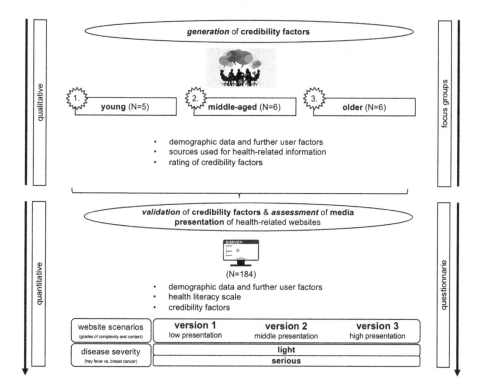

Fig. 1. Overview of research process showing both qualitative and quantitative measures to address our researach questions.

In Fig. 1, an overview of our research process is depicted. This method section is structured according to our study process. First, the results of the focus group studies are presented. Second, the development of the questionnaire will be introduced. Then the selected statistical methods and the collected samples are described.

4   Generation of Credibility Factors - The Focus Group Approach

The focus group approach aimed at gaining deeper insights into people's search behavior when looking for health related information. Moreover, the purpose was to identify and discuss people's ideas of factors which make health-related information on websites appear credible.

4.1   Method

First, participants were made familiar with the topic and the idea to gain knowledge about the individual favored kind of representation of health related information on websites. A general question (*Where do you look for health-related information?*) was raised in the beginning. Participants were encouraged to brainstorm about sources they use when informing themselves about health related information. As an "icebreaker" or rather stimulus for the discussion, the moderator shared a personal and comprehensible experience she had made recently. She described the situation of a "nervously tickling sensation" in her eye and how she started to search the Internet for reasons and for ways how to get rid of it. Thereby, she found plenty of different information partly with different opinions. Which one was she supposed to trust? In a free discussion participants started to share similar experiences. The different source types mentioned were written on paper and collected on a pin board. In a next step participants were introduced to a more serious health topic in form of a persona. Participants' were shown a picture of a mid-40-year old woman and asked to put them self in the position of the described person who just recently received a diagnosis of breast cancer. The method of the persona was intended to help the participants to identify themselves with her and start thinking from her point of view [24]. Participants were encouraged to consider where they would look for information in place of the persona. Again, all newly mentioned mediums and sources were added to the pin board. In a further step, participants were asked (*Which factors make information appear credible?*) to gather factors which make health related information on websites seem trustworthy. The mentioned factors were collected and rated due to their importance. In the end a short questionnaire was applied. Items were taken and used from related work [20] and had to be answered on a 6-point Likert scales. The duration of the focus group was about 90 min.

4.2   Sample Description

The focus group was conducted with 17 participants in total but split into three sessions. The sample was composed of 13 female and 4 male participants with an age range from 14 to 69 years ($M = 44.8$, $SD = 0.44$). One group with 5 participants was between 14 and 19 years old. The second one ($N = 6$) encompassed 30 to 54 year old participants. The third group ($N = 6$) contained 55 to 69 year old participants. The professional activities of the participants were very broadly diversified from students to employed to retired people. In general, participants have assessed themselves as very healthy with $M = 4.47$ on a six-point scale ($SD = 0.94$). The evaluation with regard to their individual health literacy turned out to be average ($M = 3.82$, $SD = 1.08$).

4.3   Results

Data of the qualitative focus group were analyzed descriptively using qualitative data analysis by Mayring [25]. Further, we used the `tidytext`, `wordcloud`, and `tm` package [26–28] to quantitatively analyze the transcripts from the focus groups in R and RStudio. Textual data was gathered from manual transcripts in pdf-files. Individual utterances were separated to allow individual-based analysis of data. Stopwords were removed using the `stopwords` package. We further removed numbers, punctuation signs, and an additional list of non-standard stopwords manually added after going through the full tokenized list. Since all transcripts of the focus groups were in German, word data was translated automatically using the Yandex-API after tokenization. All visualized data is "sanity-checked" after translation to fix possible errors of ambiguous translation. For sentiment analysis we used the SentiWS Dataset [29]. We use a bag-of-word model for sentiment analysis and manually correct for negations. We relied on this simple model of text-analysis as many of the utterances in live discussions have incoherent grammar and interjections. More advanced techniques of analysis fail to identify structure in such utterances. Therefore, we invested more effort in manual correction.

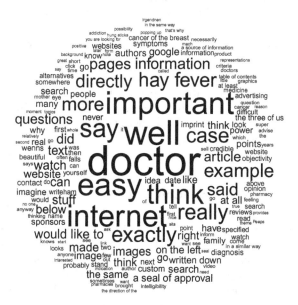

Fig. 2. Top 200 terms mentioned across all focus groups (N = 17).

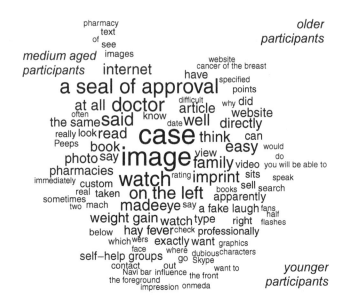

Fig. 3. Top 100 terms that were different between focus groups.

Do the Different Age Groups Differ? When we look at what the different participants mentioned during the focus groups, we see that the topics of highest interest include things like the Internet, whether one could ask questions, was there support from doctors, but also properties like easy usability, relatable examples, and images were important (see Fig. 2).

When we look at the differences between the different age groups and the topics that were relevant to the individual groups, we also see an interesting picture (see Fig. 3). While younger participants focused on ease of use and meta-data (e.g., was the date on the website shown), medium aged participants were discussing about individuality of cases, the verification of topics by doctors, inviting imagery, as well as official seals of approval. Interestingly, older participants focused their discussion around family topics, self-help groups and were mostly concerned about the imprint of a website, when it came to judging credibility.

Which Factors Make Information Appear Credible? Using correlation analysis in the term-document matrix, where documents are individual utterances, we can identify, even in a bag-of-word model what words are mentioned in conjunction frequently. Using this technique we can see, for example, what other words are mention in conjunction with the word "credible" to identify what factors influence credibility of websites. By going back to the original utterances. In Fig. 4 we see that factors such as expert opinions, certainty, experience as well as "luminaries"[1] play a role in credibility judgments.

---

[1] Participants did not mention the term "luminary", but the German word "Koryphäe", which is a relatively common word.

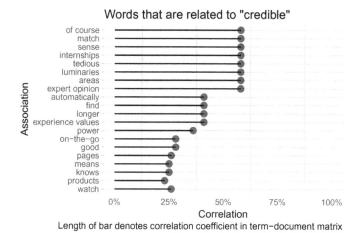

Fig. 4. Top 15 terms that were associated with the term "credible" (N = 17).

Since the use of source was stressed by the participants in many of the discussions, we wanted to see what other topics were mentioned along the term "sources" (see Fig. 5). Participants stress, when talking about sources, that comprehensibility and sources in their mother tongue (i.e., German) are helpful. Sources are used to explain and evidence and participants prefer sources where the authors are reputable scientists and doctors. Some even mentioned that video-based explanations show the quality of a website and were interested in video-conferences with doctors.

Doctors were mentioned quite a few times during the discussion. Participants were unsure whether digital information alone could ever be a solution to medical questions and wondered, whether in serious matters questions could be addressed to real doctors by email (see Fig. 6). The strategy was mostly to combine the benefits of online information with the personal relationship with a doctor. Participants are aware that going to the doctor takes time, but creates highly individualized information, but Internet search provides immediate and in-depth feedback.

Summary of Qualitative Findings. Overall, we found that scanning transcripts of focus groups using natural language processing utilities is helpful in looking for topics and relationships among topics. Still, the informal nature of such experiments creates language unfit for fully automatic evaluation and requires both manual and automatic effort. The sentiment analysis (see Table 1) requires special attention, since here a simple "not" or irony can invert the intended sentiment. But using strong sentiments as an indicator for further investigation proved helpful in finding statements, where participants made judgments about the topic at hand, which in turn were useful in factor generation. From the

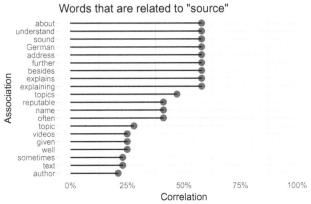

Fig. 5. Top 15 terms that were associated with the term "source" (N = 17).

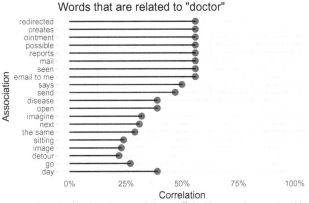

Fig. 6. Top 15 terms that were associated with the term "doctor". The term day occurs twice in the data-set due to translation (N = 17).

data we found that aspects of privacy and health literacy, but also website design and comprehensibility were important to users, focusing the research effort in the second phase of the study.

5　Validation of Credibility Factors and Media Representation - The Questionnaire Approach

To quantify the results of the focus group discussions with a larger sample, a questionnaire was developed. Results of the focus group and other criteria that can influence the credibility of health websites, such as age, gender and online privacy aspects, were taken into account and integrated into the questionnaire

Table 1. Three utterances with lowest and highest summed sentiment.

Sentiment	Text
−1.986	*"Also what, so people always like to associate all diseases they have with a symptom, I believe, and then suddenly there are totally horrible things, which are not connected at all. But someone thought hay fever now includes my stomach ache, so I'm always a bit critical about it, but..."*
−1.2836	*"Well, we only have a seal of approval because you are not sure, yes, which [sites] are there, how many and which are now right, which are not, which are faked, you don't know."*
−1.2493	*"Yes. Yes, because just really... so I never use search function, really never, therefore I did not add a point here, because most search functions are just bad on web pages I think, but I find it nevertheless somehow belongs on these websites. I don't know, normally, I would have said at the very beginning, I just do it via Google anyway."*
1.5651	*"I also think that once you have a diagnosis, you invest a lot more time in research than you do when you have a symptom and then the internet is just another good source of information. Not just the only one, I'd say, but as another source of information definitely suitable."*
0.8873	*"Yes, I have topic too, author above. Then I have text and graphics or sometimes I even like videos if they are well explained or well made. Also next to the text directly, because I think that is actually explanatory often. And I always find it very important that further topics, topics or even articles are still indicated. And at the bottom I have source and date."*
0.8429	*"That's the way I'm gonna do it. So then I look a little further and then maybe, I don't know, something serious... seems serious to me, for all I care ... on Wikipedia. Or I wouldn't look on Facebook."*

development. The survey consisted of three parts. Starting with demographic factors in part one (age, gender, education level, health status), variables regarding the person were assessed in a second part. These included the users' privacy attitudes such as privacy concerns and need for privacy. E-health literacy was also surveyed in part two. Part three examined the users' attitude concerning the different website scenarios with respect to the severity of disease. Credibility factors as generated results from the previous focus groups were also considered.

5.1   Part 1: Demographic Data and Further User Factors

The first part of the questionnaire assessed age, gender, sex, highest education level, current activity and health status. Moreover, general familiarity with the Internet usage (*For how long have you been familiar with the usage of Internet?* had to be answered on a 6-point Likert scale. The individual points were *(1) not at all, (2) less than one year, (3) 1–2 years, (4) 2–5 years or (5) 5 years and more*) as well as general Internet activities were collected (*"How much time do you weekly use for following web activities in average?"*; answering scale: no time, 0–30 min, 30–60 min, 1–2 h, 2–4 h, 4–8 h, 8 h and more). At last, usage frequency of information sources (*"How often do you use the following information sources when informing yourself about health topics?"*; answering scale: daily, 2–3 times a week, 1 time a week, monthly, 2–3 times per year, less) regarding health topics, usability of online sources (*Searching for health information, how help-*

Table 2. Items for privacy concerns, need for privacy and ehealth literacy.

	Need for privacy
(1)	Compared to others, I am less concerned about possible risks regarding my online privacy
(2)	Compared to others, I am more skeptical about what other people or businesses do with my data
(3)	Compared to others, it is more important to me that personal information about myself are kept secret
(4)	I disclose personal information to others unless they give me a reason not to do it
(5)	I have nothing to hide. That is why I feel comfortable with people who know personal thinks about me
(6)	I like to share personal information with other people and strangers
	Privacy concern
(1)	I am generally concerned about my privacy when using the Internet
(2)	I do not see any risk when leaving data behind in the Internet
(3)	I am concerned about my health data when it is collected on the Internet
	eHealth literacy
(1)	I know what health resources are available on the Internet
(2)	I know where to find helpful health resources on the Internet
(3)	I know how to find helpful health resources on the Internet
(4)	I know how to use the Internet to answer my health questions
(5)	I know how to use the health information I find on the Internet to help me
(6)	I have the skills I need to evaluate the health resources I find on the Internet
(7)	I can tell high-quality from low-quality health resources on the Internet
(8)	I feel confident in using information from the Internet to make health decisions

ful do you rate the following sources? search engines, platforms, forums, chats, websites. Each source had to be assessed on a 6-point Likert scale from 1 = not helpful at all to 6 = very helpful) as well as interest regarding health topics were assessed (*"For me, information about a healthy lifestyle/reason for cold/reason for sickness/diagnosis of cold/diagnosis of sickness/therapy of cold/therapy of sickness/medical treatment and physicians... are interesting."*.

5.2   Part 2: Need for Privacy, Privacy Concern and eHealth Literacy

Six items assessing need for privacy were taken from literature [30,31] and had to be answered on a 6-point Likert scale from 1 = I do not agree at all to 6 = I totally agree. The items are listed in Table 2.

An overall score was calculated out of the respective items after having recoded the negative items and after having checked the scale reliability (Cronbach's α = .803). Items collecting information about privacy concern were taken or adapted from different authors [30,32–35] and had to be answered on the same 6-point Likert agreement scale as above (see Table 2).

Only two items (1 & 3) reached a sufficient Alpha value with (α = .721) and were summed up to an overall score. The eHealth Literacy Scale (eHeals) by Norman and Skinner [20] was taken as an instrument that measures computer

skills with health literacy skills. In Table 2 the eight items are listed. They had
to be assessed on a 6-point Likert agreement scale.

5.3 Part 3: Website Scenarios

To find out in how far information about health topics are perceived and assessed
on websites, three existing electronic health websites were chosen by authors and
were arranged to fictive collages without naming the website brand. These developed websites could be distinguished according to its complexity of content and
preparation of site. Regarding complexity, a website was stated to be complex
when the information was more detailed and the layout contained more sub-
units. At last, one website with low content and low representation was build
(LowRep), one with a middle degree of complexity (MidRep) and a third one
with a very high complexity (HighRep). Furthermore, two diseases with different
degrees of severity were chosen. For a marginal but still serious disease hay fever
was described. Breast cancer was taken as an example for a very severe and
life striking disease. Participants were asked to look at the website leisurely and
report their impression. Therefore, they were asked to rate 5 items afterwards
on a 6-point Likert scale ($1 =$ not at all to $6 =$ yes, in any case), shown in Table 3.

Table 3. List of website assessment items.

	Website assessment items
(1)	Do you like the website?
(2)	Do you think you are sufficiently informed about the disease?
(3)	Did you perceive the website as trustworthy?
(4)	Would you still continue your search, after having seen the information?
(5)	Would you still want to see a physician, after having read the information on that website?

The articles were analyzed with regard to the different website types using a
factor analysis. Two factors have been identified. The first contained item one,
two and three, which asked about the benefits, comfort of information and credibility ($\alpha = .840$). Resulting, a scale was build and called assessment scale. The
second factor consisted of the items four and five asking about if more information is desired or a consultation with a physician is still wanted. Cronbach's
Alpha did not allow to calculate a second scale ($\alpha = .571$). Overall, 6 websites were represented; three for each disease (3 websites × 2 diseases). To avoid
fatigue effects, the order of websites was randomized.

Credibility Factors. After a "disease set", namely three website versions, the
participants were asked with which criteria a website can be classified as trustworthy. Therefore the participants had to personally name five out of 18 criteria

as being the most important ones. The choice of criteria resulted from the focus group discussion. All mentioned criteria were used here in the questionnaire for validation (e.g., publication date, source, quality seal, etc.). The whole study was run within the framework of a bachelor thesis in summer 2017 in Germany. Data was collected through the personal and professional surrounding from the candidate of the final paper as well as from the authors online and in a paper-pencil form, enabling older people to participate as well. Participation was voluntary and was not gratified. Completing the questionnaire took about 20 min.

5.4   Sample Description

Demographic Data and Further User Factors. The survey was completed by $N = 184$ participants. 40% male and 60% female participants took part in the study. The sample reached an age range between 17 and 79 years ($M = 43.5$ years, $SD = 15.7$). For an age comparison regarding different items, the sample was split by median into three age groups: 61 participants fell into the so called "digital natives" group (<29 years, 40 women and 21 men), 62 participants were assigned into the "digital immigrants" group (between 30–54 years, 37 women and 25 men) and 61 fell into the "silver surfers" group (>55 years, 33 women and 28 men). 37% of the participants hold a university degree and 29.9% a university entrance diploma. Moreover, 17.8% completed a higher education and 10.3% hold a secondary school certificate, indicating the heterogeneity of the sample's educational level. Most of the participants (36.4%) allocated their current activity in the commercial area, 19% in a technical area, 16.3% allocated it to the social field, 7.1% to a medical field, 3.3% to a artistically field and 17.9% allocated their current activity to other areas. In general, the sample constituted a rather healthy group with $M = 4.2$ ($SD = 0.85$; 6 points max.). Table 4 portrays the demographic characteristics.

Table 4. Demographic characteristics of aggregated sample (N = 184) [8].

Demographic characteristics		Percentage of respondents
Age [years]	Mean (SD)	43.5 (15.77)
	17–32 digital natives	33.2%
	33–53 digital immigrants	33.7%
	54–70 silver surfer	33.2%
Gender	Women	59.8%
	Men	40.2%
Education level	No college	61.9%
	College degree or higher	38.1%

When asked about familiarity with Internet use, the sample reported that it was quite familiar ($M = 4.93$, $SD = 0.4$). The maximum duration of Internet activities such as reading newspapers ($M = 2.53$, $SD = 1.59$), posting in news-groups ($M = 2.12$, $SD = 1.28$), receiving information about products ($M = 2.83$, $SD = 1.17$) or buying products ($M = 2.25$, $SD = 0.97$) was limited to an average duration of 0–60 min per week. When asked how often participants use certain sources for information on health topics, the Internet was most frequently use with a monthly use ($M = 4.44$, $SD = 1.21$), followed by relatives ($M = 4.44$, $SD = 1.15$). Doctors ($M = 5.06$, $SD = 0.66$), medical journals ($M = 5.49$, $SD = 0.9$) or self-help books ($M = 5.51$, $SD = 0.89$) were mentioned, which are seen or used 2–3 times a year. In addition, search engines ($M = 5.52$, $SD = 1.17$) were described as the most helpful, followed by websites ($M = 4.22$, $SD = 0.98$), platforms ($M = 3.41$, $SD = 1.24$), forums ($M = 3.12$, $SD = 1.21$) and recent chats ($M = 2.44$, $SD = 1.09$). It was also of interest what kind of informa-tion the participants were looking for on the Internet. Information on a healthy lifestyle ($M = 4.13$, $SD = 1.22$) followed by information on the treatment of serious diseases ($M = 3.85$, $SD = 1.17$). Information on medical treatments ($M = 3.85$, $SD = 1.26$) and doctors ($M = 3.75$, $SD = 1.4$) were reported before causes ($M = 3.79$, $SD = 1.22$) or diagnosis of diseases ($M = 3.61$, $SD = 1.26$). The least important search terms among the health information were given due to a cold ($M = 2.6$, $SD = 1.27$) and a cold diagnosis ($M = 2.49$, $SD = 1.14$).

Need for Privacy and Privacy Concerns. The participants reported that they were a little concerned about their privacy ($M = 3.93$, $SD = 0.76$). The results on the need for privacy scale reflect similar results with $M = 2.82$ ($SD = 0.61$). A significant age difference was observed in the privacy concern attitude ($F(2, 170) = 6.19; p = 0.003$). Here, older participants showed the high-est concern regarding their online privacy and disclosure of health data with a mean of $M = 4.10/6$ points max. ($SD = 0.83$) in contrast to the youngest group with a mean of $M = 3.66/6$ points max. ($SD = 0.73$).

e-Health Literacy. The health literacy level was averagely high with $M = 3.84$ ($SD = 0.79$). In this context, a significant age ($F(2, 152) = 4.01; p = 0.020$) and gender ($F(1, 152) = 5.05; p = 0.026$) effect could be detected. The ability to search, find, read, understand and evaluate health information from electronic sources was rated significantly higher by the youngest group ($M = 4.06$, $SD = 0.7$) than by the oldest group ($M = 3.59$, $SD = 0.85$). Female participants ($M = 3.96$, $SD = 0.87$) rated their competence to evaluate digital health information higher than male ($M = 3.67$, $SD = 0.63$) participants.

5.5   Results

All subjective measures were evaluated on six-point Likert scales. The data were analyzed quantitatively using Pearson correlations, ANOVA with repeated mea-surement and MANOVA. The level of significance was set to $\alpha = .05$. This means that significant findings can occur in 1 out of 20 such studies, even if the effect is not present.

5.6   Validation of Credibility Factors

The presentation of the results is guided by the research questions and is structured as follows: First, findings concerning the credibility factors of a health information website are presented. Secondly, the assessment of websites types (low, middle, high) regarding its complexity and its content (light disease vs. serious disease) will be outlined. The section closes with findings about the impact of user diversity regarding the assessment of websites.

Factors Influencing Credibility. In order to identify credibility factors that affect recipients' attitudes to rating a website with health information as trustworthy, participants had to identify five out of 18 criteria that were rated as personally most important. As most important comprehensibility was mentioned, followed by objectivity of the information, clear structure of the website reference and the indication of negative side effects or risks. Factors with low credibility were links to other websites, access to forums or chat rooms or images of authors. Considering the severity of diseases, the picture is different. Table 5 shows the results. If one compares the five most frequently mentioned credibility factors of a mild and a severe disease, it turns out that four aspects are the same only with a different significance. For example, comprehensibility is assessed as the most important aspect of health-related information for both sides. Other factors mentioned differ due to the severity of the disease. While the clarity of a website plays the second most important role for the health-related information of a mild disease, objectivity is mentioned in the second step. Level five contains information on authors as a credibility factor for a mild disease. In contrast, the date of publication is assessed as another important credibility factor for the digital health information of a serious disease. Taking into account the three different age groups, the factors mentioned remain the same, only the order of the factors mentioned differs slightly.

Table 5. Five most important assessed credibility factors of health-related websites with different disease contexts in % (N = 184) [8].

Light disease	in %	Severe disease	in %
Comprehensibility	64.7	Comprehensibility	62.0
Clarity	54.3	Objectivity	48.4
Objectivity	49.5	References	46.2
References	39.7	Clarity	39.7
Details about author	29.9	Date of publication	33.2

Assessment of Different Websites. In order to find out to what extent the media presentation of a health website and the severity of the disease play a role in the user's assessment, a repeated measure was calculated. Looking only at the media presentation of all three websites without the content of diseases, no significant difference could be found $(F(1.82, 300.57) = 2.57, p = .084)$. Nevertheless, the most complex version was rated best $(M = 3.49, SD = 0.77)$, followed by the second complex version $(M = 3.44, SD = 0.78)$ and finally the version with the least complexity $(M = 3.34, SD = 0.88)$. Interestingly, significant differences were found including the different severity of the diseases $(F(3.7, 581.5) = 5.75, p < .01)$. Since Mauchly's test showed that the assumption of sphericity was violated $(\chi^2(14) = 113.48, p < .01)$, the Greenhouse Geisser corrected tests are reported $(=.74)$. For the less severe disease version two achieved the best rating $(M = 3.64, SD = 0.87)$. In contrast, of the three different website versions, version three was rated best for the more life-threatening disease $(M = 3.44, SD = 0.9)$.

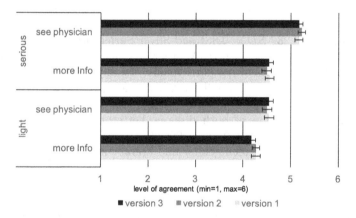

Fig. 7. Assessment of website regarding if more information is wished for and if a physician wants to be seen after having seen website. Error-bars denote standard error [8].

The results suggest that evaluating the complexity of websites always plays an important role when describing a particular disease. More serious diseases are preferably read on the most complex website, as opposed to a mild disease. In our case, the participants liked to read information about a mild illness in a more unusual way. Significant results were also found $(F(4.42, 680.15) = 25.72, p < .01)$ when asked whether, after seeing the website together with the nature of the disease, participants would like to seek further information or see a doctor. Figure 7 shows the different characteristics. The desire to get more information and to see a doctor increases with the severity of the disease. The evaluation of website versions shows a different picture. The most complex website seems to provide better information in the case of a mild illness than in the case of a serious illness in contrast to the other versions. However, the less complex website versions one and two seem to provide satisfactory information about the more serious disease than about a mild one. The same result can be seen at the article, if a doctor would like to be consulted afterwards. The less complex websites seem to represent trustworthy information. In summary it can be said that at first glance the severity of the disease plays an important role, but small differences between the disease and the website version could be determined.

5.7 Impact of User Diversity on Assessment of Websites

In order to investigate to what extent user factors such as age, gender, health status or health competence influence the assessment of health information of varying degrees of severity, a MANOVA was carried out. The health status and the literacy variable were divided into three equal groups. The results show that three significant interactions have been found between gender and assessment, age and health. Women rated the least complex mild disease presentation better than men ($F(1, 113) = 5,997$, $p = .016$/Female $= 3.39$, $SD = 0.93$; Male $= 3.23$, $SD = 0.92$). The least complex presentation of the serious disease was rated better by Digital Natives ($M = 3.81$, $SD = 1.14$) than by Digital Immigrants ($M = 3.23$, $SD = 0.88$) and Silver Surfer ($M = 3.13$, $SD = 0.77$) with $F(2, 113) = 4.915$, $p = .009$. Another significant result was found with regard to the health status of the participants. Usually participants with a better state of health (values for mild illness Version: $M_{bestHealth} = 3.57$, $SD = 0.7$; $M_{middleHealth} = 3.25$, $SD = 0.86$; $M_{badHealth} = 2.75$, $SD = 0.85$) rated the least complex presentation of both diseases better than not so healthy people ($F_{lightdisease}(2, 113) = 5.382$, $p = .006$/$F_{severedisease}(2, 113) = 4.443$, $p = .019$). Two interactions between gender and literacy as well as age and literacy have been identified. The first interaction was observed in the assessment of the least complex presentation of both diseases ($F_{lightDisease}(2, 113) = 5,579$, $p = .005$ and $F_{severeDisease}(2, 113) = 3,854$, $p = .024$). Women with significantly higher health literacy rated the website version better than men with comparatively low health literacy. The results regarding the mild and severe disease are very similar. Due to the spatial limitations of this article, only one finding according to the mild disease is shown in Fig. 8.

Another interaction can be reported on age and eHealth literacy in relation to the most complex website presentation and mild disease ($F(4, 113) = 2,655$, $p = .037$). As can be seen in Fig. 9, the youngest age group with a high eHealth competence value rated the most complex website version better than the middle and older age group.

6 Discussion and Guidelines

Discussion. "In clarity we trust!" sums up one important credibility factor that affects the recipients' attitude of trusting a health website in our study. We will discuss this aspect as well as further results of our study in this section. We wanted to understand which elements on a website with health-related information convince or rather satisfy people to trust health-related information. Therefore, we conducted a study with two objectives: first of all, we examined factors from websites with health information that trigger credibility. Secondly,

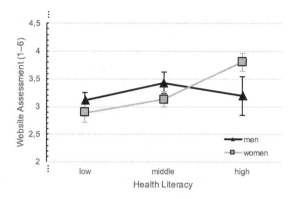

Fig. 8. Interaction of gender and eHealth literacy (low, middle, high) regarding assessment of least complex presentation of light disease. Error bars denote standard error [8].

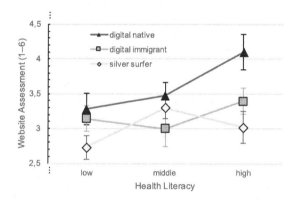

Fig. 9. Interaction of three age-groups (digital native, digital immigrant and silver surfer) and eHealth literacy (low, middle, high) regarding assessment of least complex presentation of light disease. Error bars denote standard error [8].

we examined to what extent both the media presentation of health websites and the severity of the disease play a role in assessing credibility. Last but not least, we took a look at the nature of eHealth literacy as well as privacy concerns considering general search behavior. To do so, we chose a two-way multi method approach. That way, we could gather more robust results and deal with the complexity of research question in detail. In a first step, focus groups were run, in which we analyzed users' search behavior when looking for health-related information and collected people's ideas of factors which make health-related information on websites appear credible.

In a second step, an online questionnaire was sent out in which the results of the focus groups were quantified as well as how digital health information is judged by its recipient and how it varies with the severity of the disease. Findings were analyzed with a diversity focus, thus comparing gender and age groups with respect to media representation, severity of disease, eHealth literacy, and privacy concerns. Insights won from the focus group study show that users, in general, look for a number of factors when deciding whether the information is trustworthy (see Table 5). The factors range from content factors to layout factors. Comprehensibility and sources written in their mother tongue were stressed. User attach importance to understandable and prepared information. Another aspect relates to a clear information structure. A clear structure guides the users and gives them confidence in handling the information. The objectivity of the information is another credibility aspect. Information that conveys a neutral position is more accepted than subjective descriptions of health details. Among the five most important trustworthy elements, source references were also cited. Information about the sources is also considered important. What's more, users want to know more about the authors' details. In this respect, our results are consistent with those of Eysenbach and Köhler [13].

When looking to the outcomes in the questionnaire study, again, it was corroborated that users independent of age or gender attach high importance to comprehensibility and clarity as an important credibility element. In our study it was of additional interest to what extent aspects that trigger trustworthiness of information differ for diseases of varying severity. It turns out that the type of factors remains the same, only the order of priorities varies. Comprehensibility remains the most important aspect. While factors such as clarity trigger trustworthiness in the case of a mild disease, objectivity is more important in the case of a more severe disease. Another difference we found was that details about authors are of interest when they inform themselves about a mild disease (in this case hay fever) compared to the publication date, which triggers credibility in the search for a more life-threatening disease. In the latter case, patients have a stronger urge to stay up to date and to not overlook the latest advances in therapy.

One focus of our research was directed to the media presentation of health-related websites. To find out to what extent information on health topics is perceived and evaluated on websites, we have selected three existing electronic health websites and compiled them into fictitious collages without naming the website brand. These developed websites could be distinguished according to their complexity and presentation. In terms of complexity, a website was considered more complex if the information was more detailed and the layout contained more sub-units. It is interesting to note that differences in the perception of credibility are not only due to differences in information complexity. There are no differences in the evaluation when a simple comparison of the means compares their evaluations. Only if user factors or the type of disease are taken into account, differences occur. For instance, gender-sensitive differences could be found when looking at websites with low content and low representation (LowRep) of a mild disease. Women gave a higher rating than men. Moreover, women distinguished themselves with a higher literacy compared to men in regard to assessing a "LowRep" website. It seems that women in general assign a different search and rating pattern than men in this context [23]. Not only gender but also age and health status seem to play an important role when it comes to assessing websites. Younger people seem to be rather satisfied with information of "LowRep" websites than older. The same result turned out for healthy people. However, people with a lower health status seem to have a different point of view regarding the complexity of websites. They rate more complex websites better. This might occur from the fact that people who are less healthy and thus might be more desperate to find solutions to their health problems rather trust well designed websites which are easy to read and understand [23].

We have learned from this study regarding the findings of eHealth literacy and privacy concerns, that people differ in their privacy attitudes when searching for online information. Awareness of data sharing and possible consequences seems to occupy older users more than younger ones. This may be due to the fact that older people are generally not as familiar with Internet applications as are younger people [36]. Thus, older people seem to be more skeptical about Internet activities. This aspect is also reflected in the results in terms of health literacy. Younger participants show a higher competence to evaluate and judge information on the Internet.

Guidelines. Our results show that websites that try to inform the public about health issues must take their information and communication concept into account. In relation to our website evaluation, these results mean that there does not seem to be a "one-size-fits-all" solution when it comes to health information on the Internet. Information providers should be aware of how to design websites for different target groups and possibly consider participatory design methods to determine who needs which information, when, and how. As there are systematic differences in judgments based on health literacy, gender and age, these factors should not be ignored when designing a health-related website. It is important to understand the target group and its health information requirements. Adaptable websites that allow users to seamlessly increase the complexity of a particular disease without hindering clear and easy access to information could provide a solution to such challenges. In this context, the use of a health-conscious recommendation system [37] could be used to determine the information needs of the user depending on the interaction on the website [38]. When other users interact with information in forums or comments, additional, non-verified information enters the stage. In such health-related social media, some users are more active than others [39]. Information and above all meta-information can "drift" through user interaction - especially when algorithms determine the presentation of information (e.g., through evaluation, sympathy). The integration of human oversight into doctor-in-the-loop approaches could be interesting [40].

6.1 Limitations and Future Research

Limitations. As with any empirical study, our results are subject to limitations. The interaction effects studied are suitable for a relatively small subgroups of participants. For example, the older male participants with high health competence are a rather small subgroup of users. This is shown by the size of the larger error bars in the illustrations. Nevertheless, there are effects even with higher error margins. Since our results are consistent with previous studies, further confirmation and transferability of the results would require significantly larger samples or meta-analytical methods to improve evidence.

Since the settings were generated from fictitious websites created by the authors, we cannot be sure that our view of the complexity is shared equally by all users. We have tried to design the websites in such a way that the complexity increases in "equidistant" steps. However, since the texts and images we use come from actual websites, it is not easy to guarantee this. The diseases selected by us (hay fever, breast cancer) have very specific target groups. Men who participated in the study found it difficult for them to put themselves in an environment that required breast cancer therapy. Although men could in fact develop breast cancer, it was strongly regarded as a women's disease. Furthermore, the question in this study was raised exclusively in healthy participants. At this point, it would be of interest to subject the same research question to a sample with ill participants; especially, on the assumption that personal involvement has an impact on the evaluation of health-related information [16]. As with all scenario-based questionnaires, all results must be taken up with a grain of salt, as the social distortion of desirability could more distort the answers in a more alien environment for the participant.

Future Research. Questions of ethics, data protection [41], and trust naturally play an important role in such solutions we discussed in the guidelines. What information are users willing to share to improve their online experience on health-related websites? Diversity factors play an even greater role here [42]. Therefore, it is necessary to understand the interaction of all user-related factors and the benefits that users see when using such websites. By modelling benefits and privacy, better services or mobile phone applications can be designed with better information quality. The presentation and complexity of these services are adapted to the needs and wishes of users, also taking into account their current usage context. Are you looking for help or just browsing? Should they trust the information they find or should they see a doctor? Either way, the factors that determine the credibility of health information are crucial to help patients, both online on the Internet and offline through a doctor.

Acknowledgements. We thank all participants for their participation and their willingness to share their thoughts and opinions. Furthermore, the research support of Jenny Reinhard is highly acknowledged. This research has been funded by the German Ministry of Education and Research (BMBF) under the project Whistle.

References

1. Fischer, F., Dockweiler, C.: Qualität von onlinebasierter Gesundheitskommunikation. In: Fischer, F., Krämer, A. (eds.) eHealth in Deutschland, pp. 407–419. Springer, Heidelberg (2016). https://doi.org/10.1007/978-3-662-49504-9_22
2. Andreassen, H.K., et al.: European citizens' use of e-health services: a study of seven countries. BMC Publ. Health **7**, 53 (2007)
3. Trepte, S., Baumann, E., Hautzinger, N., Siegert, G.: Qualität gesundheitsbezogener online-angebote aus sicht von usern und experten. M&K Medien & Kommunikationswissenschaft **53**, 486–506 (2005)
4. Cline, R.J., Haynes, K.M.: Consumer health information seeking on the internet: the state of the art. Health Educ. Res. **16**, 671–692 (2001)
5. Eysenbach, G., Kohler, C.: What is the prevalence of health-related searches on the world wide web? Qualitative and quantitative analysis of search engine queries on the internet. In: AMIA Annual Symposium Proceedings, vol. 2003, p. 225. American Medical Informatics Association (2003)
6. Dierks, M., Lerch, M., Mieth, I., Schwarz, G., Schwartz, F.: Wie können Patienten gute von schlechten Informationen unterscheiden? Der Urologe B **42**, 30–34 (2002)
7. Kim, P., Eng, T.R., Deering, M.J., Maxfield, A.: Published criteria for evaluating health related web sites. BMJ **318**, 647–649 (1999)
8. Vervier, L., Calero Valdez, A., Ziefle, M.: "Should I trust or should I go?" Or what makes health-related websites appear trustworthy? In: Proceedings of the 4th International Conference on ICT for Ageing Well (2018)
9. Medlock, S., et al.: Health information–seeking behavior of seniors who use the internet: a survey. J. Med. Internet Res. **17**(1) (2015)
10. Kienhues, D., Stadtler, M., Bromme, R.: Dealing with conflicting or consistent medical information on the web: when expert information breeds laypersons' doubts about experts. Learn. Instr. **21**, 193–204 (2011)
11. Wilson, P.: How to find the good and avoid the bad or ugly: a short guide to tools for rating quality of health information on the internet. BMJ: Br. Med. J. **324**, 598 (2002)
12. Fahy, E., Hardikar, R., Fox, A., Mackay, S.: Quality of patient health information on the internet: reviewing a complex and evolving landscape. Aust. Med. J. **7**, 24 (2014)
13. Eysenbach, G., Köhler, C.: How do consumers search for and appraise health information on the world wide web? Qualitative study using focus groups, usability tests, and in-depth interviews. BMJ **324**, 573–577 (2002)
14. Bates, B.R., Romina, S., Ahmed, R., Hopson, D.: The effect of source credibility on consumers' perceptions of the quality of health information on the internet. Med. Inform. Internet Med. **31**, 45–52 (2006)
15. Benigeri, M., Pluye, P.: Shortcomings of health information on the internet. Health Promot. Int. **18**, 381–386 (2003)
16. Barnes, M.D., et al.: Measuring the relevance of evaluation criteria among health information seekers on the internet. J. Health Psychol. **8**, 71–82 (2003)
17. Fogg, B.J., Soohoo, C., Danielson, D.R., Marable, L., Stanford, J., Tauber, E.R.: How do users evaluate the credibility of web sites?: a study with over 2,500 participants. In: Proceedings of Conference on Designing for User Experiences, pp. 1–15. ACM (2003)
18. Huntington, P., Nicholas, D., Gunter, B., Russell, C., Withey, R., Polydoratou, P.: Consumer trust in health information on the web. In: ASLIB Proceedings, vol. 56, pp. 373–382. Emerald Group Publishing Limited, Bingley (2004)

19. Nutbeam, D.: The evolving concept of health literacy. Soc. Sci. Med. **67**, 2072–2078 (2008)
20. Norman, C.D., Skinner, H.A.: eHEALS: the eHealth literacy scale. J. Med. Internet Res. **8**(4) (2006)
21. Paasche-Orlow, M.K., Wolf, M.S.: The causal pathways linking health literacy to health outcomes. Am. J. Health Behav. **31**, S19–S26 (2007)
22. Morahan-Martin, J.M.: How internet users find, evaluate, and use online health information: a cross-cultural review. Cyberpsychol. Behav. **7**, 497–510 (2004)
23. Cotten, S.R., Gupta, S.S.: Characteristics of online and offline health information seekers and factors that discriminate between them. Soc. Sci. Med. **59**, 1795–1806 (2004)
24. Pruitt, J., Grudin, J.: Personas: practice and theory. In: Proceedings of the 2003 Conference on Designing for User Experiences, pp. 1–15. ACM (2003)
25. Mayring, P.: Qualitative inhaltsanalyse. In: Mey, G., Mruck, K. (eds.) Handbuch Qualitative Forschung in der Psychologie, pp. 601–613. Springer, Heidelberg (2010). https://doi.org/10.1007/978-3-531-92052-8_42
26. Silge, J., Robinson, D.: tidytext: Text mining and analysis using tidy data principles in R. JOSS **1**, 37 (2016)
27. Fellows, I.: wordcloud: Word Clouds (2014)
28. Feinerer, I., Hornik, K., Meyer, D.: Text mining infrastructure in R. J. Stat. Softw. **25**, 1–54 (2008)
29. Remus, R., Quasthoff, U., Heyer, G.: SentiWS - a publicly available German-language resource for sentiment analysis. In: LREC (2010)
30. Xu, H., Dinev, T., Smith, H.J., Hart, P.: Examining the formation of individual's privacy concerns: toward an integrative view. In: ICIS 2008 Proceedings, p. 6 (2008)
31. Morton, A.: Measuring inherent privacy concern and desire for privacy - a pilot survey study of an instrument to measure dispositional privacy concern. In: 2013 International Conference on Social Computing (SocialCom), pp. 468–477. IEEE (2013)
32. Joinson, A., Piwek, L.: Technology and the formation of socially positive behaviours. In: Beyond Behaviour Change: Key Issues, Interdisciplinary Approaches and Future Directions, p. 157 (2016)
33. Li, Y.: The impact of disposition to privacy, website reputation and website familiarity on information privacy concerns. Decis. Support Syst. **57**, 343–354 (2014)
34. Kehr, F., Wentzel, D., Mayer, P.: Rethinking the privacy calculus: on the role of dispositional factors and affect. In: Thirty Fourth International Conference on Information Systems (ICIS 2013). AIS Association for Information Systems (2013)
35. Dinev, T., Xu, H., Smith, H.J.: Information privacy values, beliefs and attitudes: an empirical analysis of web 2.0 privacy. In: 42nd Hawaii International Conference on System Sciences, HICSS 2009, pp. 1–10. IEEE (2009)
36. Prensky, M.: Digital natives, digital immigrants. Horizon **9**, 1–6 (2001)
37. Schäfer, H., et al.: Towards health (aware) recommender systems. In: Proceedings of International Conference on Digital Health, pp. 157–161. ACM (2017)
38. Calero Valdez, A., Ziefle, M., Verbert, K., Felfernig, A., Holzinger, A.: Recommender systems for health informatics: state-of-the-art and future perspectives. In: Holzinger, A. (ed.) Machine Learning for Health Informatics. LNCS (LNAI), vol. 9605, pp. 391–414. Springer, Cham (2016). https://doi.org/10.1007/978-3-319-50478-0_20
39. Schaar, A.K., Calero Valdez, A., Ziefle, M.: Social media for the eHealth context. a requirement assessment. In: Advances in Human Aspects of Healthcare, p. 79 (2012)

40. Holzinger, A., Calero Valdez, A., Ziefle, M.: Towards interactive recommender systems with the doctor-in-the-loop. In: Mensch und Computer-Workshopband (2016)
41. Vervier, L., Zeissig, E.M., Lidynia, C., Ziefle, M.: Perceptions of digital footprints and the value of privacy. In: Proceedings of IoTBD 2017, pp. 80–91 (2017)
42. Zeissig, E.-M., Lidynia, C., Vervier, L., Gadeib, A., Ziefle, M.: Online privacy perceptions of older adults. In: Zhou, J., Salvendy, G. (eds.) ITAP 2017. LNCS, vol. 10298, pp. 181–200. Springer, Cham (2017). https://doi.org/10.1007/978-3-319-58536-9_16

Extending Exergame-Based Physical Activity for Older Adults: The e-Coaching Approach for Increased Adherence

Despoina Petsani[1], Evdokimos I. Kostantinidis[1], Unai Diaz-Orueta[2],
Louise Hopper[3], and Panagiotis D. Bamidis[1(✉)]

[1] Lab of Medical Physics, Medical School, Aristotle University of Thessaloniki,
Thessaloniki, Greece
`despoinapets@gmail.com`, `evdokimosk@gmail.com`,
`bamidis@auth.gr`
[2] Department of Psychology, Maynooth University, Maynooth, Ireland
`unai.diazorueta@mu.ie`
[3] School of Nursing and Human Sciences, Dublin City University,
Dublin, Ireland
`louise.hopper@dcu.ie`

Abstract. e-Coaching approaches have recently received a lot of attention, as technology led healthy ageing solutions depend on empowering older people's motivation. While the beneficial impact of physical activity for older populations is indisputable, this work aims at presenting first designing considerations to be followed if increased adherence to physical activity through an e-coaching system were to be aimed for older adults. The work plan kicks-off on the basis of an existing exergame platform, especially designed and widely tested for older adults (webFitForAll) which is forced to align with notion of behavior change techniques (BCTs) that have been developed for physical activity enhancement. New advances in micro-projector technologies provide extra opportunities for tweaking the accessibility burden while augmenting and blending the real with the coaching environment. Quite reasonably, these are not easy tasks to follow and success depends much on multi-disciplinary approaches encompassing new ideas from co-creation and co-design with the actual users.

Keywords: e-Coaching · Physical activity · Exergames · Older adults

1 Introduction

In recent years the value of shifting from instructing and patronizing a person during her daily exercise to coaching and helping towards making own choices is indisputable. It is crucial to encourage motivation and empowerment in adapting to lifelong changes and enable older people to co-design their everyday exercise plan. To this extent, coaching has been defined as an ongoing process of self-enhancement and effective goal striving with the observation, aid and collaborative conversation with an expert, referred as coach [1].

P. D. Bamidis et al. (Eds.): ICT4AWE 2018, CCIS 982, pp. 108–125, 2019.
https://doi.org/10.1007/978-3-030-15736-4_6

Furthermore, necessity of the digitalization of various functions in a wide variety of domains, including coaching practices is emerging both in industry and academia. The necessary components for an automatic, digital coaching system are to be ubiquitous, individualized, constantly adapting and gathering information while providing the necessary feedback. Besides the irreplaceable need for human-to-human interaction, the financial cost and the human resources needed may be dissuasive. The broader penetration of technology in our everyday life may increase the acceptance of non-human coaches, while advances in technology could provide ways to include the presence of human coaches in digital systems like e-coaching.

The term e-coaching is mostly utilized in literature for systems that are used to enable communication with human coaches [2, 3]. However, the term should not refer to systems that facilitate or conceptualize the coaching, but to systems that do the coaching (nonhuman coaches).

An explicit definition of what an e-coaching system is, together with the key-elements it must include, is considered timely and necessary to effectively develop any e-coaching environment. As Kamphorst [4] states, the e-coaching system must have a sufficient level of sophistication and independence and defines the e-coaching system as "a set of computerized components that constitutes an artificial entity that can observe, reason about, learn from and predict a user's behaviours, in context and over time [...]" [4, p. 5]. This definition underlines some key-points for e-coaching systems, which must be:

- context-aware [1, 5]
- personalized
- capable of collecting information from the user (direct or other measurements)
- able to forecast and plan future steps.

The use of virtual coaching for the support of physical activity in later life have increased in the latest years. Dikhuis et al. [6] proposed a personalized and flexible machine-learning-based procedure to automate a part of the coaching process and serve as a source of information on a participant's progress with physical activity during the day, providing information on the probability of the participant meeting his or her daily physical activity goal. Albaina et al. [7] found that integrating a virtual coach was influential in establishing trust and confidence towards the system leading to favorable outcomes. In their study with the Flowie virtual coach, they found that those using a virtual coach felt motivated to exercise more, while other studies lacking these features led to increase dropouts.

This paper extends the authors' previous work [8] in which an e-coaching system for promoting physical activity for older population, expanding an already existing exergaming platform was proposed. Three major points are covered herein, including (a) the importance of physical activity for older people with a focus on positive impacts of physical exercise on cognitive function; (b) a revisit to behavior change techniques (BCTs) that have been developed for physical activity enhancement; (c) the formulation of designing goals/guidelines for the future implementation of a proposed e-coaching system.

2 Physical Activity in Older Populations

With the constant growth of aging population, the concept of active and healthy aging has become a serious socioeconomic concern. According to the World Health Organization (WHO) physical activity plays a decisive role in maintaining or achieving a good quality of life (QoL) [9]. Many positive effects have been associated with regular physical activity including reduced risks of developing Alzheimer's disease (AD) [10], osteoporosis [11] or cardiovascular disease [12]. Moreover, a great cohort of studies have pointed out the positive impact of physical exercise on psychology, functional capacity, autonomy and general QoL [13–16].

Epidemiological studies [17] show that lifestyle factors such as physical exercise significantly decrease the risk to develop cognitive decline associated to dementia or AD. With regards to physical activity and development of dementia, according to a study in Canada with more than 9,000 male and female subjects, moderate levels of physical exercise may reduce up to a 40% the risk for cognitive decline and subsequent development of AD [18–20]. Different researchers have showed that a moderate level of aerobic physical activity is likely to improve cognitive and brain function and decelerate or even revert neural decline frequently observed in older adults [23], while other have reviewed the associated neuroscientific evidence of such interventions [21] In terms of activity duration, some studies obtain visible results and significant improvements from 2 to 6 months of intervention [22–24],. Some factors have been proposed as explanatory mechanisms for the protective effect of physical activity in cognition, such as decreased level of cardiovascular risk and metabolic syndrome by means of an improvement of cerebral perfusion, angiogenesis, capillarization, and modulation of neurotrophic factors such as the Brain Derived Neurotrophic Factor (BDNF) [25, 26] as well as an increase of neurogenesis and hippocampal neurotrophic factors, thereby providing with improvements in cognitive functions and learning; or the preservation of the integrity of the white matter that comes from and reaches to prefrontal regions [21, 23].

In terms of the type of exercise, there is evidence in favour of the association between aerobic exercise and a structural and functional increase in regions of the frontal and temporal cortex associated to age-related decline. Kramer [27] point out that it is possible that physical activities are more strongly related with cognition than anaerobic activities, mainly with measures of executive control (planning, working memory, inhibitory processes and performance of different tasks simultaneously). Moreover, effects of physical activity seem to be larger when aerobic training programmes are combined with anaerobic training for strength and flexibility [23].

The most notorious beneficial effects from physical exercise are those related to frontal, parietal and temporal regions, which are critical for high level cognitive functions. In this sense, many studies have shown the relationship between physical activity and learning abilities [28–33] due to the fact that physical exercise stimulates the secretion of BDNF [34] thus improving synaptic connections. BDNF provides life support for cholinergic neurons of the anterior cortex, which is related to the neurodegeneration caused by AD. Thus, higher levels of inducted BDNF thanks to physical exercise may help increase resistance to injury and neurodegeneration.

Moreover, BDNF may be a mediator for the improvement of cerebral plasticity and appears to be highly related to learning and memory development. Finally, while in healthy ageing the relationship between physical activity and health seems to be clear, the relation between physical activity and AD is not that clear, though some studies such as the one by Scarmeas [35] have shown that a combination of a Mediterranean diet and high levels of physical activity may lead to decreased risks for AD.

2.1 Attitudes and Motivation Towards Physical Activity Among Older Adults

Although the positive effects of physical activity in health are well established, older adults tend to face cessation of physical activity as an inevitable consequence of aging. A majority of older adults confront exercise as a waste of time that often perceived to have negative effects on their body (sweating, muscle soreness, etc.) [34] while about 50% of exercise intervention participants tend to drop out before realizing any health benefits [35]. According to Picorelli et al. [36], benefits of exercise depend on continued participation, but, in case of older adults, the concurrence of higher co-morbidity, less social support, and more disability and depression than the general population, may become factors associated with lower exercise adherence. Moreover, especially with older populations, it is essential to understand the individual, social, community and demographic factors associated with adherence to physical activity. In relation to this, Picorelli et al. [36] found that factors associated with greater adherence include higher socioeconomic status, living alone, better health status, better physical ability, better cognitive ability and fewer depressive symptoms.

It is here where an e-coaching system may be helpful to provide the motivation and guidance needed. In terms of motivation for exercise, Eyck et al. [37] remind us that in psychology, two types of motivation are distinguished: intrinsic and extrinsic. Intrinsic motivation is related to the satisfaction a person gets from an activity, whereas extrinsically motivated activities are done to receive rewards, under pressure or to avoid punishment. Previous research gathered by these authors have shown that intrinsic motivation is a very important determinant for exercise adherence, but mixed results have been achieved with regards to the effect of a virtual coach on this intrinsic motivation, with results for dimensions such as perceived control and usefulness but not for the most important of all (i.e. enjoyment).

Any technology-based coach aiming at promoting physical activity and lifestyle changes may also need to keep in mind what is known as persuasive strategies. According to Khaghani et al. [38], persuasive strategies for home-based training can be grouped in two major categories:

1. Individual: strategies that leverage the individual wills and natural drive, and,
2. Social: strategies that demand the presence of a community of people with the roles of family, supporters and peer trainees.

This links with the work of Fogg [39], who describes a series of strategies that could be relevant for home-based training applications by means of, for example, a virtual coach:

- Individual Persuasion Strategies
  - Positive & negative reinforcement: The application prompts positive or negative feedback about the exercising behavior of participants.
  - Rewards: The application praises the participant by providing virtual prizes, such as medals, awards and recognition upon completion or success on exercising sessions.
  - Reminders and suggestions: The application reminds participants of their exercises sessions and suggests better habits.
  - Self-monitoring: The application provides to participants, performance monitoring and awareness about their current progress.
- Social Persuasion Strategies
  - Social learning (observation of others and comparison), cooperation and competition: The fitness app provides social features that allow participants to compare their performance with others, cooperate to achieve common objectives, or, on the contrary, to compete against each other.
  - Social support: The application provides social features such as messaging and shared forums that enable participants to discuss, talk to each other and create a community of people supporting each other.
  - Recognition: The participants, both on an individual and group basis, get public recognition on their awards, progress and contributions.

Recently, Mohadis et al. [40] performed a review on the existing persuasive devices for promoting physical activity. In their review, they confirm the central role of self-efficacy for the prediction of attitudes and behavior towards physical activity, with different studies linking higher levels of physical activity with higher self-efficacy and a better physical functional performance. In terms of the social components linked to activity, they found that people with high self-efficacy are more likely to be active if they have social support, but, in contrast, people with low self-efficacy were less likely to be physically active, even if they had social support. Among the reasons for a perception of a low self-efficacy, we could find poor health and lack of physical abilities, and this low self-efficacy does not improve (actually, it may go worse) with the inclusion of social learning and comparison with others.

According to Dikhuis et al. [6], in order to improve physical activity in combination with activity trackers, a coaching feature will be relevant and helpful only when three main factors are kept in mind: personalization, context and timing. Perceiving the coaching information as personal and relevant is crucial for the effectiveness of e-coaching. Moreover, timeliness of information is important for participants to be able to process the information and apply the advice while it is still relevant for them, something that will be achieved by means of accessing to real-time predictions. This kind of individually personalized models for e-coaching could help both the coach and the participant in the process of behavior change and increased physical activity.

Environmental factors may also restrain older adults' devotion to physical activity more than younger people. To give an example, older people will avoid walking outside when it is raining or snowing. Social or economic barriers are also reported [36]. E-coaching system should provide appealing and low-cost alternatives for exercise regardless of social and environmental restrictions.

2.2 Physical Activity Guidelines

Taking into account the e-coaching system key-points mentioned above, the context and the target group have to be carefully studied in order to elucidate specific needs and barriers. The recommended levels of physical activity for older adults as reported by the academic community are presented to gather context and user group aware information. The Center for Disease Control and Prevention (CDC) proposed that levels of activity should meet the individual abilities of the person, avoiding inactivity [41]. The minimum suggested activity by CDC for achieving health benefits is 150 min of moderate-intensity aerobic activity or 75 min of vigorous-intensity aerobic activity and muscle strengthening activities for all muscle groups on at least two days of the week. The American College of Sports Medicine (ACSM) has also suggested at least two days per week strength exercises to improve flexibility and balance [16].

Aerobic activities may include bicycle, dancing, walking or jogging, swimming, tennis etc. [42]. Muscle strengthening activities may also be simulated by carrying groceries, pilates, washing windows or the floor, some activities of gardening, etc.

2.3 The webFitForAll Exergaming Platform

A few years ago, during the Long Lasting Memories EC project (www.longlasting-memories.eu), attempts to gamify and digitalize physical exercise led to the creation of an exergame platform that encapsulated the necessary amount of exercise in an attractive way for older adults [15, 43] easily configured to address personalized plan for each participant. The first version of the platform, FitForAll (FFA) was widely tested and exhibited significant results in improving the Quality of Life (QoL) and physical condition of older users [15].

This platform was later expanded with the use of proper web technologies as well as open, ontological descriptions of exercises under the brand name webFitForAll (wFFA) game platform [44]. wFFA is a true web based serious game platform specially designed for older adults. wFFA includes physical exercises and games that promote physical activity and contribute in advance and maintenance of wellbeing and QoL. It has achieved high acceptability rates for its participants, as well as significant improvements in participants' bodily capacity and fitness [45]. Each session is composed of aerobic, strength, balance and flexibility exercises designed in a playful, simple and understandable way and lasts about 60 min. The participant can achieve the guidelines threshold of physical activity per week if engaged for a minimum of three times.

wFFA is connected with a depth sensor camera which supports two functionalities: (i) the user interaction with the system with his/her body movement and posture. In that way the user-computer interaction is simpler and no prior knowledge of computer usage is required (ii) the system records and stores user's body part movements for further analysis.

3 Behavior Change Techniques Implementation in the e-Coaching System

As mentioned above, e-coaching systems support an ongoing process and effort to achieve a goal, improve or change a situation. It is critical for the design of these systems to focus on the inclusion of BCTs so as to be effective. Systems using persuasive strategies have been shown to be effective in establishing and maintaining healthy habits including interventions through physical activity [46–48]. However, in order for these systems to support effective behavior changes, they must be adapted to the specific requirement of the target behavior and to the particular needs and preferences of the target user groups [49, 50]. Although the importance of inclusion of BCTs

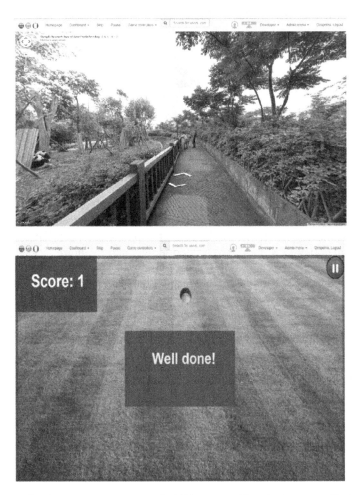

Fig. 1. Example of two wFFA games. In the hiking game (above), the user walks in a Google Street View environment according to his/her body posture and steps. In the golf game (below) the user moves a ball according to his/her body movement, trying to put it in the hole [8].

is undeniable, the majority of e-coaching systems lack examination and adjustment of that technique with specific populations including older adults [47, 51]. Furthermore, many existing persuasive systems have demonstrated poorer results for older adults than for younger adults [52]. As a result, it is essential to enrich e-Coaching systems aimed at older adults with additional BCTs capacities that have been shown to facilitate effective behavior changes within such target groups [53, 54].

3.1 Proposed Taxonomy of Behavior Change Techniques

Michie [55] have defined a taxonomy (the CALO-RE) that enables identification, categorization and understanding of 40 BCTs that lead to effective behavioral intervention including those for physical activity behaviors. Persuasive systems generally incorporate BCTs relating to goal setting, identification of discrepancies between current and target behavior, feedback and self-monitoring, and social support [56, 57]. A systematic review has identified three additional BCTs that are particularly effective in changing physical activity levels in older adults, namely 'provide rewards contingent on successful behavior', 'barrier identification or problem solving' and 'model or demonstrate the behavior' [52].

The BCTs of the proposed e-coaching system will be designed in 3 phases: the starting, the design and adaptation and the intervention phase. The design and intervention phases are not strictly segregated as the design phase could re-implemented through the intervention. Figure 2 shows the timeline of the 3 phases and dependencies and relations between them. Barriers and motivators for change can arise in each of these phases [58].

In the starting phase, the readiness and motivation for change should be assessed and enhanced. In assessing willingness to change, it is critical to improve self-regulatory skills in those adults most at risk of developing adherence issues [59]. The main challenge in this phase is for the e-coach to support the individual's exploration of their own physical activity levels and adequately answer the question "Why changing my physical activity routine if I currently function satisfactorily?" For this reason, the system has to provide evidence-based information about the impact that the upcoming intervention will have for the individual. Information about the general approval of the system, the behaviour of other groups and the reliability must also be reported. In this way, the e-coaching system is incorporating the BCTs 'model or demonstrate the behavior' and 'barrier identification or problem solving'.

The behavior and overall outcome goals are clarified in the design phase. Here, the main effort is personalizing the intervention. The system and the user must agree the actions that have to be taken paying special attention to the environmental, socioeconomic and individual barriers each individual may face. This information is stored for possible readjustment of the behavior plan. The active participation of the individual in this phase ensures that the goals and associated tasks are realistic and cognizant of each person's abilities. The user, in our case the older adult, will make a behavioral "contract" that they accept the designed plan and will commit to it. This may be in form of formal consent with the system or a selected familiar person [60].

The intervention phase is where behavior change happens. The personalized intervention is based on the plan agreed in the previous phase. To retain adherence, the system must reward the participant for achieving goals or for making progress. Older adults have expressed a need for feedback that acknowledges the specific effort they have made towards their goals, but that also praises them for having been active, thus highlighting the importance of the BCT 'provide rewards contingent on successful behavior' [49]. Rewards can include collecting points that are shared among a groups' members that go through similar intervention, using the same e-coaching system. The e-coaching system facilitates and plans this social support based on the participant's desire and encourage social comparison. However, the reward must be proportionate to the progress and each time an anticipation must be created for future rewards. Hence, progress measurement must be reliable and meaningful to the individual [49]. Feedback is also provided for each separate task, along with suggestions and demonstrations on how to achieve better results. The ability to adapt previously set plans is a key component of any coaching system and the e-coach must observe, question, tailor, agree and adapt plans as needed in order to maximize adherence [61]. Feedback and instruction must be simple, clear, and supported with audiovisual content as the user must both receive and understand the persuasive message in order for attitude and behavior change to take place. Personal interest and motivation must remain high [54]. For older adults, effective stress and time management is also beneficial for successful health outcomes [62].

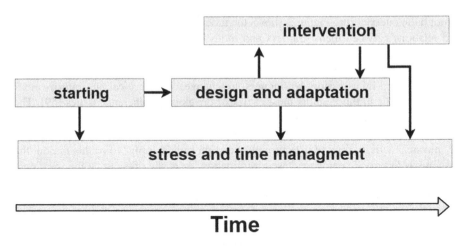

Fig. 2. Timeline of the proposed coaching intervention strategy.

Another important point is to define an exit strategy. This is not considered as a part of the e-coaching procedure, therefore it is not included in the e-coaching phases. If a user decides to stop the intervention or the system detects a long-term abstention from his/her weekly schedule, the exit strategy has to be enabled. Throughout this phase, the primary input is the reasons that lead the user to this decision. Also, the system presents the current state of the procedure and the user's progress so far and reminds him/her of the initial commitment and the possible benefits. If the user insists on quitting a short questionnaire about the reasons for this decision is delivered to him/her.

3.2   BCTs Implementation

As mentioned above, the wFFA platform has been well-established. However, to fit the e-coaching system approach and deliver a complete e-coaching system for increased adherence of physical activity in older populations, additional components and changes have to be implemented.

In the starting phase the system should exhibit the benefits of wFFA, related to physical condition and overall QoL, as derived from wide pilot deployments. wFFA maintains a database of interventions that were carried out among different vulnerable populations groups. More precisely, the system compares the user's profile and presents charts and images of the progress of people with similar profiles in the database. These data are supplemented by real statements of participants for the effect of the platform use in their physical exercise and the overall impression to increase reliability. General statistics for the value of physical exercise for older populations are also presented in a comprehensive way e.g. charts and images and more personalized content, deriving from literature, based on user's health condition is provided. For example, for older adults with Parkinson's disease the information about the benefits of exercising will focus on relative literature findings for Parkinson's and not general population. The information must be presented in a comprehensive and intuitive way to keep user's interest unchanged.

wFFA exergame platform consists of a default protocol of four levels with different difficulties and also provides the option to modify each session manually. Each level differs in terms of intensity and requires more physical and cognitive effort as well as increased attention. The design phase's main goal is to individualize the sessions of wFFA based on the overall goal and participant's preferences. To this extend, the e-coaching system should also motivate the user to do physical activities besides wFFA, based on her/his character and other environmental issues that can limit such activities. For instance, the user can agree to take a walk outside instead of the hiking game of wFFA (Fig. 1) once a week. The system should also provide individualized proposal for recreational activities located near home, for instance yoga lessons in the near park. Moreover, activities of daily living (e.g. carrying groceries) could have equivalent effects with muscle strengthening exercise. To this extend, special attention should be paid to include these activities in the weekly physical activity plan. The user must be able to indicate such activities during the week and the system should replace other scheduled activities.

Each game in the wFFA platform is preceded by visual instructions (video) accompanied by a simple text (Fig. 3). During the game, the participant collects points e.g. number of balls in the hole (Fig. 1). In addition, a scoring functionality has been designed and is under development. A score for each game will be calculated depending on the data collected during users' interaction with the system. wFFA correlates in-game metrics (users' gaming performance measurements) with neuropsychological assessment tests of previous users and compares them with the current users to produce a meaningful score that reflects the actual improvement in the physical and cognitive domains [63].

Due to its web-based implementation, wFFA can easily support social interaction between users. Researches have shown that many activity behaviors have been determined by social environmental characteristics [64]. wFFA will be extended to a social media platform, user-friendly designed for older adults where they can connect with other people using the platform. The achievement of a goal or the augment of a score will be shared among desired users to promote competition. Also, the user can challenge his/her digital friends to gather more points or play a game simultaneously.

Finally, the system would provide additional instructions during the exercises execution, correcting body posture and other mistakes. Body posture is easily recognized by the depth sensor camera used in wFFA platform interaction. The appropriate movements in each game and exercise have been configured by health care professionals and physicians.

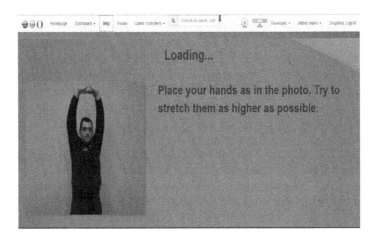

Fig. 3. Visual and text instructions before an exercise [8].

4   Designing the e-Coaching Environment

Two aspects should be considered when designing the framework of an e-coaching environment: what are the suggestions that the system would do and how these should be addressed to the user. The former is based on option generation techniques and effective counseling dialogue system development, while the latter is about defining the most appropriate interface and information gathering technique, taking into consideration the target group, in this case older populations.

The proposed options, about what a system must propose, exhibit two probable implications. On one hand, they can influence the decision making process and impact the final decision [39]. Coaching is an ongoing process supported by implementation of BCTs, so it is possible to intervene with people's decision. Consequently, the system's suggestions must be carefully planned. On the other hand, repeatedly suggestions and indications that a person rejects, may harm system's reliability. The proposals must in general agree with what a person consider as an option and be contingent on his character [65]. The system must produce a dialogue explaining its importance of a rejected suggestion and make appropriate questions to identify the reasons of its rejection. The additional information concerning the rejection will help the system learn more about user's character. In case an option is accepted and successfully carried out, the system encourages and praises the accomplishment. An holistic dialogue ontology is an absolute necessity to support counseling and enhancement of physical activity, taking into consideration the specific needs of older adults.

Regarding the appropriate way to provide information (the how), vision impairment and reduction of precision in motor skills should be taken into account as a frequently encountered consequence of aging. These difficulties can prevent older adults from using conventional computer interfaces like mouse, keyboard, small buttons or gestures requiring slick movements. User interfaces aimed at older adults must be clean, friendly and not include redundant material. These are included to the key issues that are defined as: usability, acceptability and reliability, meaning that the participant can easily interact with the technology, accept it in their everyday life and gain confidence that the system effectively interacts with him/her.

An innovative technology that incorporates the three keys issues, is augmented reality through projections. The system could project contextualized information, wherever and whenever needed, without the use of external devices like mobile phones or tablets. The user-system interaction is accomplished by touching or moving actual objects, without the need of specific skills or preexisting knowledge. The e-coaching environment, therefore, complements or even better augments the real-life environment, thereby increasing its acceptability chances for older adults. Furthermore, the interactions allowed in real life movements, with absence of buttons or touch screens could eliminate the stress of pushing the "wrong" button [66].

In the wFFA platform, the system is controlled by user's movement. The system captures the necessary information from a 3D depth sensor camera that detects human body joints. The graphic information is presented in a computer screen. Projections can replace computer screens in future implementations so that the system blends in the users' home environment without distracting them.

Moreover, a speech UI will be implemented, providing another one simple and clean interaction with the system. There is a great amount of available API's for speech to text transform that can utilized for speech recognition (e.g. Google Assistant, Amazon Alexa, IBM Watson). After the speech commands have been transferred to text, the text output will be fed to the dialogue component. The outputs of the dialogue component will be again transform into speech and be given to the user as an audio reply.

Finally, user monitoring is a component of vital importance for an e-coaching system. Behavioral, physiological as well as emotional information about the user is important to be gathered. This can be done unobtrusively with the use of 3D sensing systems that have already exhibited a great amount of applications, including facial image technologies to capture emotional states, gait analysis, communication with traditional devices like blood pressure meters and pulse oximeters (NFC or Bluetooth solutions) and physical and cognitive state indicators through serious games in-game metrics [63].

5   Discussion

The current work has discussed some of the key issues in e-coaching systems with emphasis on increased adherence to physical activity for older adults. To achieve a first implementation of such a system, the already existing wFFA exergame platform is employed, but ideally expanded to align with the notions of BCT and the augmented environments and interfaces brought about by new advancements such as those of micro-projectors (Fig. 4).

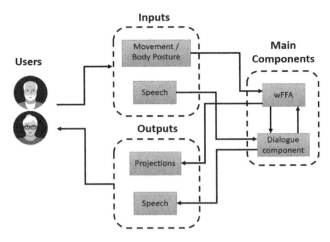

Fig. 4. The e-coaching system components, voice interface and movement monitoring.

Successful health coaching encompasses more than just measureable goals and activities. It includes the promotion of health behaviors, enhanced health literacy, and motivational support that not only promotes health behaviors but also leads to increased self-efficacy for the user. The more personalized the intervention and the advice, the more likely the system users are to adhere to their improvement plans and experience sustainable health behavior changes. It is indisputable that e-coaching systems can add value by building on the ability of ICT to embed validated health behavior interventions into a coaching relationship, by incorporating high quality prompts, motivators, and feedback, and by simplifying and personalizing the end user experience [58]. The ultimate goal is the intrinsic motivation of the users such that they are best placed to achieve their specific short-term goals which in turn enhances their self-efficacy and motivates them to continue on the path to healthy behavioral change. The question that arise is when the intervention is considered successful and how we can evaluate that the user is now able to continue his/her physical activity routine without the system's support.

An issue that raises questions about e-coaching systems is the exclusion of human specialists. The presented design aims at the inclusion of human therapists/doctors or a familiar person chosen by the user who can have access to the stored data. The real challenge is to give an active role to human factors (family, friends and healthcare professionals) so as to improve the coaching process [67]. Active engagement of human factor includes not only the supervision of the stored data but also an advisory, supporting and inspiring role.

Future work will also include focus groups, meeting and interviews with older adults in order to gain an insight about their needs and preferences. A first goal is to understand the reasons why older adults tend to abstain from physical exercise despite the undeniable benefit for their health. Furthermore, it is crucial to capture their point of view about possible motivation to exercise. These will enrich our approach with new techniques for increased adherence. The proposed UI will also be tested. Before the real implementation and integration with the wFFA platform, a working prototype will be created. The prototype included the functionalities of the UI but not the full implementation of the system. That way the users can understand how the real system will produce the output information and are able to provide valuable feedback and new suggestions.

In conclusion, the construction of an e-coaching system must not be confronted with naivety. The design challenge extends beyond the mere ICT domain as the development of a successful persuasive e-Coaching system will demand co-creation and co-design with end users, and the embedding of persuasive strategies and BCTs appropriate to the population of interest. Therefore, it is a complex process that demands a multidisciplinary approach including psychology, computer science, medical science and engaged citizens.

References

1. Ives, Y.: What is 'coaching'? An exploration of conflicting paradigms. Int. J. Evid. Based Coach. Mentor. **6**(2), 100–113 (2008)
2. Boratto, L., Carta, S., Mulas, F., Pilloni, P.: An e-coaching ecosystem: design and effectiveness analysis of the engagement of remote coaching on athletes. Pers. Ubiquitous Comput. **21**(4), 689–704 (2017)
3. Allen, M., Iezzoni, L.I., Huang, A., Huang, L., Leveille, S.G.: Improving patient-clinician communication about chronic conditions: description of an internet-based nurse e-coach intervention. Nurs. Res. **57**(2), 107–112 (2008)
4. Kamphorst, B.A.: E-coaching systems: what they are, and what they aren't. Pers. Ubiquitous Comput. **21**(4), 625–632 (2017)
5. Pecora, F., Cirillo, M., Dell'Osa, F., Ullberg, J., Saffiotti, A.: A constraint-based approach for proactive, context-aware human support. J. Ambient Intell. Smart Environ. **4**(4), 347–367 (2012)
6. Dijkhuis, T.B., Blaauw, F.J., van Ittersum, M.W., Velthuijsen, H., Aiello, M.: Personalized physical activity coaching: a machine learning approach. Sensors (Switzerland) **18**(2), 623 (2018)
7. Albaina, I.M., Visser, T., van der Mast, C.A.P.G., Vastenburg, M.H.: Flowie: a persuasive virtual coach to motivate elderly individuals to walk. In: Proceedings of the 3D International ICST Conference on Pervasive Computing Technologies for Healthcare (2009)
8. Petsani, D., Konstantinidis, E.I., Bamidis, P.D.: Designing an e-coaching system for older people to increase adherence to exergame-based physical activity. In: Proceedings of the 4th International Conference on Information and Communication Technologies for Ageing Well and E-Health, ICT4AWE, pp. 258–263 (2018)

9. World Health Organization: Recomendaciones Mundiales sobre Actividad Física para la Salud, Geneva WHO Library Catalog Number. Completo, pp. 1–58 (2010)
10. Laurin, D., Verreault, R., Lindsay, J., MacPherson, K., Rockwood, K.: Physical activity and risk of cognitive impairment and dementia in elderly persons. Archiv. Neurol. **58**(3), 498–504 (2001)
11. Nguyen, T.V., Center, J.R., Eisman, J.A.: Osteoporosis in elderly men and women: effects of dietary calcium, physical activity, and body mass index. J. Bone Miner. Res. **15**(2), 322–331 (2000)
12. Geffken, D.F., Cushman, M., Burke, G.L., Polak, J.F., Sakkinen, P.A., Tracy, R.P.: Association between physical activity and markers of inflammation in a healthy elderly population. Am. J. Epidemiol. **153**(3), 242–250 (2001)
13. Taguchi, N., Higaki, Y., Inoue, S., Kimura, H., Tanaka, K.: Effects of a 12-month multicomponent exercise program on physical performance, daily physical activity, and quality of life in very elderly people with minor disabilities: an intervention study. J. Epidemiol. **20**(1), 21–29 (2010)
14. Vagetti, G.C., Barbosa Filho, V.C., Moreira, N.B., de Oliveira, V., Mazzardo, O., de Campos, W.: Association between physical activity and quality of life in the elderly: a systematic review, 2000–2012. Rev. Bras. Psiquiatr. **36**(1), 76–88 (2014)
15. Konstantinidis, E.I., Billis, A.S., Mouzakidis, C.A., Zilidou, V.I., Antoniou, P.E., Bamidis, P.D.: Design, implementation, and wide pilot deployment of FitForAll: an easy to use exergaming platform improving physical fitness and life quality of senior citizens. IEEE J. Biomed. Health Inform. **20**(1), 189–200 (2016)
16. Chodzko-Zajko, W.J., et al.: Exercise and physical activity for older adults. Med. Sci. Sports Exerc. **41**(7), 1510–1530 (2009)
17. Yaffe, K., et al.: Predictors of maintaining cognitive function in older adults. Neurology **72**, 2029–2035 (2009)
18. Larson, E.B., et al.: Exercise is associated with reduced risk for incident dementia among persons 65 years of age and older. Ann. Intern. Med. **144**(2), 73–81 (2006)
19. Lytle, M.E., Vander Bilt, J., Pandav, R.S., Dodge, H.H., Ganguli, M.: Exercise level and cognitive decline: the MoVIES project. Alzheimer Dis. Assoc. Disord. **18**(2), 57–64 (2004)
20. Podewils, L.J., et al.: Physical activity, APOE genotype, and dementia risk: findings from the cardiovascular health cognition study. Am. J. Epidemiol. **161**(7), 639–651 (2005)
21. Bamidis, P.D., et al.: Review: a review of physical and cognitive interventions in aging. Neurosci. Biobehav. Rev. **44**, 206–220 (2014). Applied Neuroscience: Models, methods, theories, reviews. A Society of Applied Neuroscience (SAN) special issue
22. Colcombe, S.J., et al.: Aerobic exercise training increases brain volume in aging humans. J. Gerontol. Ser. A Biol. Sci. Med. Sci. **61**(11), 1166–1170 (2006)
23. Erickson, K.I., Kramer, A.F.: Aerobic exercise effects on cognitive and neural plasticity in older adults. Br. J. Sports Med. **43**(1), 22–24 (2009)
24. Bamidis, P.D., et al.: Gains in cognition through combined cognitive and physical training: the role of training dosage and severity of neurocognitive disorder. Front. Aging Neurosci. **7**, 152 (2015)
25. Etgen, T., Sander, D., Huntgeburth, U., Poppert, H., Förstl, H., Bickel, H.: Physical activity and incident cognitive impairment in elderly persons: the INVADE study. Arch. Intern. Med. **170**(2), 186–193 (2010)
26. Liu-Ambrose, T., et al.: Promotion of the mind through exercise (PROMoTE): a proof-of-concept randomized controlled trial of aerobic exercise training in older adults with vascular cognitive impairment. BMC Neurol. **10**(1), 14 (2010)
27. Kramer, A.F.: Exercise, cognition, and the aging brain. J. Appl. Physiol. **101**(4), 1237–1242 (2006)

28. Barde, Y.A.: Neurotrophins: a family of proteins supporting the survival of neurons. Prog. Clin. Biol. Res. **390**, 45–56 (1994)
29. van Praag, H., Christie, B.R., Sejnowski, T.J., Gage, F.H.: Running enhances neurogenesis, learning, and long-term potentiation in mice. Proc. Natl. Acad. Sci. **96**(23), 13427–13431 (1999)
30. Berchtold, N.C., Kesslak, J.P., Cotman, C.W.: Hippocampal brain-derived neurotrophic factor gene regulation by exercise and the medial septum. J. Neurosci. Res. **68**(5), 511–521 (2002)
31. Cotman, C.W., Berchtold, N.C.: Exercise: a behavioral intervention to enhance brain health and plasticity. Trends Neurosci. **25**(6), 295–301 (2002)
32. Cotman, C.W., et al.: Exercise enhances and protects brain function. Exerc. Sport Sci. Rev. **30**(2), 75–79 (2002)
33. Russo-Neustadt, A., Ha, T., Ramirez, R., Kesslak, J.P.: Physical activity-antidepressant treatment combination: impact on brain-derived neurotrophic factor and behavior in an animal model. Behav. Brain Res. **120**(1), 87–95 (2001)
34. Fissler, P., Küster, O., Schlee, W., Kolassa, I.T.: Novelty interventions to enhance broad cognitive abilities and prevent dementia: synergistic approaches for the facilitation of positive plastic change. Prog. Brain Res. **207**, 403–434 (2013)
35. Scarmeas, N., et al.: Physical activity, diet, and risk of Alzheimer disease. JAMA **302**(6), 627 (2009)
36. Picorelli, A.M.A., Pereira, L.S.M., Pereira, D.S., Felício, D., Sherrington, C.: Adherence to exercise programs for older people is influenced by program characteristics and personal factors: a systematic review. J. Physiother. **60**(3), 151–156 (2014)
37. Eyck, A., et al.: Effect of a virtual coach on athletes' motivation. In: IJsselsteijn, W.A., de Kort, Y.A.W., Midden, C., Eggen, B., van den Hoven, E. (eds.) PERSUASIVE 2006. LNCS, vol. 3962, pp. 158–161. Springer, Heidelberg (2006). https://doi.org/10.1007/11755494_22
38. Khaghani-Far, I., Nikitina, S., Baez, M., Taran, E.A., Casati, F.: Fitness applications for home-based training. IEEE Pervasive Comput. **15**(4), 56–65 (2016)
39. Fogg, B.J.: Persuasive technology: using computers to change what we think and do. Ubiquity **2002**(December) (2002). https://doi.org/10.1145/764008.763957
40. Mohadis, H.M., Mohamad Ali, N., Smeaton, A.F.: Designing a persuasive physical activity application for older workers: understanding end-user perceptions. Behav. Inf. Technol. **35**(12), 1102–1114 (2016)
41. CDC: How much physical activity do adults need?—Physical Activity—CDC. Center for Disease Control and Prevention (2015)
42. U.S. Department of Health and Human Services: 2008 Physical activity guidelines for Americans. Pres. Counc. Phys. Fit. Sport. Res. Dig. **9**(4), 1–8 (2008)
43. Bamidis, P.D., et al.: A Web services-based exergaming platform for senior citizens: the long lasting memories project approach to e-health care. In: Proceedings of the Annual International Conference of the IEEE Engineering in Medicine and Biology Society, EMBS, pp. 2505–2509 (2011)
44. Konstantinidis, E.I., Bamparopoulos, G., Bamidis, P.D.: Moving real exergaming engines on the web: the webFitForAll case study in an active and healthy ageing living lab environment. IEEE J. Biomed. Heal. Inform. **21**(3), 859–866 (2017)
45. Zilidou, V.I., Konstantinidis, E.I., Romanopoulou, E.D., Karagianni, M., Kartsidis, P., Bamidis, P.D.: Investigating the effectiveness of physical training through exergames: focus on balance and aerobic protocols. In: Proceedings of TISHW 2016 - 1st International Conference on Technology and Innovation in Sports, Health and Wellbeing (2016)

46. Matthews, J., Win, K.T., Oinas-Kukkonen, H., Freeman, M.: Persuasive technology in mobile applications promoting physical activity: a systematic review. J. Med. Syst. **40**(3), 1–13 (2016)
47. Orji, R., Moffatt, K.: Persuasive technology for health and wellness: state-of-the-art and emerging trends. Health Inform. J. **24**, 1–26 (2016)
48. Sanders, J.P., et al.: Devices for self-monitoring sedentary time or physical activity: a scoping review. J. Med. Internet Res. **18**(5), e90 (2016)
49. Ehn, M., Eriksson, L.C., Åkerberg, N., Johansson, A.-C.: Activity monitors as support for older persons' physical activity in daily life: qualitative study of the users' experiences. JMIR mHealth uHealth **6**(2), e34 (2018)
50. Fisk, A.D., Rogers, W.A., Charness, N., Czaja, S.J., Sharit, J.: Designing for Older Adults: Principles and Creative Human Factors Approaches, p. 176. CRC Press, Boca Raton (2009)
51. Mollee, J.S., Middelweerd, A., Kurvers, R.L., Klein, M.C.A.: What technological features are used in smartphone apps that promote physical activity? A review and content analysis. Pers. Ubiquitous Comput. **21**(4), 633–643 (2017)
52. French, D.P., Olander, E.K., Chisholm, A., Mc Sharry, J.: Which behaviour change techniques are most effective at increasing older adults' self-efficacy and physical activity behaviour? A systematic review. Ann. Behav. Med. **48**(2), 225–234 (2014)
53. Mercer, K., Li, M., Giangregorio, L., Burns, C., Grindrod, K.: Behavior change techniques present in wearable activity trackers: a critical analysis. JMIR mHealth uHealth **4**(2), e40 (2016)
54. Patel, M.S., Asch, D.A., Volpp, K.G.: Wearable devices as facilitators, not drivers, of health behavior change. JAMA - J. Am. Med. Assoc. **313**(5), 459–460 (2015)
55. Michie, S., Ashford, S., Sniehotta, F.F., Dombrowski, S.U., Bishop, A., French, D.P.: A refined taxonomy of behaviour change techniques to help people change their physical activity and healthy eating behaviours: the CALO-RE taxonomy. Psychol. Health **26**(11), 1479–1498 (2011)
56. Lyons, E.J., Swartz, M.C., Lewis, Z.H., Martinez, E., Jennings, K.: Feasibility and acceptability of a wearable technology physical activity intervention with telephone counseling for mid-aged and older adults: a randomized controlled pilot trial. JMIR mHealth uHealth **5**(3), e28 (2017)
57. Stephenson, A., McDonough, S.M., Murphy, M.H., Nugent, C.D., Mair, J.L.: Using computer, mobile and wearable technology enhanced interventions to reduce sedentary behaviour: a systematic review and meta-analysis. Int. J. Behav. Nutr. Phys. Act. **14**(1), 105 (2017)
58. Simons, L.P.A., Hampe, J.F., Guldemond, N.A.: ICT supported healthy lifestyle interventions: design lessons. Electron. Mark. **24**(3), 179–192 (2014)
59. Culos-Reed, S.N., Rejeski, W.J., McAuley, E., Ockene, J.K., Roter, D.L.: Predictors of adherence to behavior change interventions in the elderly. Control. Clin. Trials **21**(5), S200–S205 (2000)
60. Michie, S., Abraham, C., Whittington, C., McAteer, J., Gupta, S.: Effective techniques in healthy eating and physical activity interventions: a meta-regression. Health Psychol. **28**(6), 690–701 (2009)
61. Beun, R.J., et al.: Improving adherence in automated e-coaching. In: Meschtscherjakov, A., De Ruyter, B., Fuchsberger, V., Murer, M., Tscheligi, M. (eds.) PERSUASIVE 2016. LNCS, vol. 9638, pp. 276–287. Springer, Cham (2016). https://doi.org/10.1007/978-3-319-31510-2_24
62. Abraham, C., Michie, S.: A taxonomy of behavior change techniques used in interventions. Health Psychol. **27**(3), 379–387 (2008)

63. Petsani, D., Kostantinidis, E.I., Zilidou, V.I., Bamidis, P.D: Creating health profiles from physical and cognitive serious game analytics. In: International Conference on Technology and Innovation in Sports, Health and Wellbeing, TISHW 2018 (2018)

64. McNeill, L.H., Kreuter, M.W., Subramanian, S.V.: Social environment and physical activity: a review of concepts and evidence. Soc. Sci. Med. **63**(4), 1011–1022 (1982). https://doi.org/10.1016/j.socscimed.2006.03.012reuter

65. Kamphorst, B., Kalis, A.: Why option generation matters for the design of autonomous e-coaching systems. AI Soc. **30**(1), 77–88 (2014)

66. Steele, R., Lo, A., Secombe, C., Wong, Y.K.: Elderly persons' perception and acceptance of using wireless sensor networks to assist healthcare. Int. J. Med. Inform. **78**(12), 788–801 (2009)

67. Geissler, H., Hasenbein, M., Kanatouri, S., Wegener, R.: E-coaching: conceptual and empirical findings of a virtual coaching programme. Int. J. Evid. Based Coach. Mentor. **12**(2), 165–186 (2014)

Vision-Based Marker-Less Spatiotemporal Gait Analysis by Using a Mobile Platform: Preliminary Validation

Benjamin Filtjens[1,2,5(✉)], Robin Amsters[2,5], Ali Bin Junaid[2,5], Nick Damen[5], Jeroen Van De Laer[5], Benedicte Vanwanseele[3,6], Bart Vanrumste[1,4], and Peter Slaets[2,5]

[1] eMedia Research Lab, KU Leuven, 3000 Leuven, Belgium
{benjamin.filtjens,bart.vanrumste}@kuleuven.be
[2] Intelligent Mobile Platform Research Group, KU Leuven, 3000 Leuven, Belgium
{robin.amsters,ali.binjunaid,peter.slaets}@kuleuven.be
[3] Human Movement Biomechanics Research Group, KU Leuven,
3001 Heverlee, Belgium
benedicte.vanwanseele@kuleuven.be
[4] Department of Electrical Engineering (ESAT), STADIUS - IMEC, KU Leuven,
3001 Heverlee, Belgium
[5] Department of Mechanical Engineering, KU Leuven, 3001 Heverlee, Belgium
{nick.damen,jeroen.vandelaer}@kuleuven.be
[6] Department of Movement Sciences, KU Leuven, 3001 Heverlee, Belgium

Abstract. Gait analysis is one of the most useful tools for assessing age-related conditions. This study describes the preliminary validation of a novel vision-based method for unobtrusive, ambulatory monitoring of spatiotemporal gait parameters. The method uses a mobile platform that is equipped with a Microsoft Kinect. A proprietary, generative tracker is used for measuring the 3D segmental movement of the subject. A novel method was developed for extracting gait parameters from the raw joint measurements by using the relative distance between the two ankle joints. The results are assessed in terms of mean absolute error and mean absolute percentage error with respect to a motion capture system. The mean absolute error ± precision was 5.5 ± 3.5 cm for stride length, 1.7 ± 1.3 cm for step width, 0.93 ± 0.44 steps/min for cadence, and 2.5 ± 2.0% for single limb support. While these results are promising, additional experiments are required to assess the repeatability of this approach.

Keywords: Marker-less · Spatiotemporal · Gait analysis · Mobile platform · Robot · Kinect · Kalman

1 Introduction

Europe is experiencing unprecedented demographic changes characterized by rapid ageing and workforce decline. In 1950, only 12% of the European population was over 65. Today, this share has already doubled, and projections show

© Springer Nature Switzerland AG 2019
P. D. Bamidis et al. (Eds.): ICT4AWE 2018, CCIS 982, pp. 126–141, 2019.
https://doi.org/10.1007/978-3-030-15736-4_7

that in 2050 over 36% of Europe's population will be over 65 years old [1]. So how will the next generations deliver appropriate care, despite the increasing demand on healthcare related services by older persons and a decline of the working population? These statistics suggest that healthcare needs a shift towards more scalable and affordable solutions. Personalized healthcare has emerged as a concept to address these challenges, focusing on prevention and early detection of age related conditions, and treatment options tailor-made for individuals [2]. In Europe, implementing personalized medicine has been recognized in the conclusions of the Council of the European Union at its meeting on 7 December 2015 and through funding programs such as Horizon 2020 [3,4]. With social and assistive robots becoming a useful addition in the care for older adults [5,6], a logical next step is to extend their functionality by incorporating modules to monitor important health indicators. Mobile robots may then also become a key technology in providing continuous, ambulatory monitoring. In this paper, a module is presented for ambulatory monitoring of a person's gait, one of the most important health indicators, with predictors for three of the most common long-term care admittance factors [7] such as cognitive impairment [8], Parkinson's disease (PD) [9], and functional decline [10]. Gait analysis is thus not only useful to assess a person's general motor performance, but also to assess the progression of ageing and age-related conditions. For example, PD is typically characterized by severe, unpredictable changes of the patient's motor functioning that fluctuate markedly over the course of a day [11]. The assessment of these fluctuations, which determines the therapeutic intervention, is difficult and relies on a subjective patient diary and on clinical scales such as the Unified Parkinson Disease Rating Scale [12], which has limited assessment of a person's gait [9]. An objective long-term ambulatory measurement may provide more effective treatment assessment, and possibly a more accurate diagnosis of PD [11]. Targeted interventions have proven successful in decreasing the severity of the conditions. However, identifying a population of people who would most benefit from an intervention is a tedious and difficult process. Thus, not only has ambulatory monitoring proven useful in the assessment and prediction of the severity of the disease, it can also help identify people who would most benefit from an intervention.

Despite these advantages, there has been limited use of gait analysis in daily clinical practice, caused by the inherent difficulty of measuring human motion. The most widely used standard for gait analysis, a gait laboratory consisting of a multi infra-red camera array that records the movement of reflective markers, allows for accurate and complete gait analysis. This method, however, requires a dedicated lab, has long set-up times, and is thus very expensive. Furthermore, it assumes that gait in an imposed path and time is representative of usual gait performance, yet a significant mismatch has been noted between movement measured in a laboratory and movement measured ambulatory, attributed to dual tasking gait with another cognitive activity [13] and the influence of being monitored [14]. Therefore, this method has limited applicability in assessing a person's regular gait and is thus used almost exclusively for research, with clinical use limited to assessing surgical outcomes [15]. In comparison, a mobile robot can closely monitor an individual's changes in his or her gait and provide feedback to help maintain an optimal health status. In addition, patients can benefit from continuous monitoring as part of a rehabilitation process, providing optimal feedback to the therapist about the efficacy of the treatment. Furthermore, autonomous ambulatory monitoring provides personalized feedback about a patient, allowing screening of patients that would most benefit with treatment.

2   Related Work

A comprehensive review of all methods related to gait analysis is outside the scope of this article, for this information we refer the reader to the following list of recent articles on motion capture methods [16,17] (markerless, respectively marker-based), wearable devices [18,19], pressure sensors [20], and observational methods [21]. This section will instead focus on methods with the potential to be used ambulatory, which is defined as the continuous observation of free-moving subjects in everyday life [22]. The concept of ambulatory measurement of gait is not new, dating back as far as 1878 [23]. More recent ambulatory systems can be subdivided into three categories: foot switches and pressure sensors, wearable devices, and single camera vision-based methods.

Foot switches [24] and pressure insoles [25] work by attaching sensors to the sole of the foot. These methods provide high reliability in evaluating gait phases and normal walking behaviour. However, problems such as mechanical failure and the inability to detect shuffling gait limit their applicability [26]. Therefore, these methods are mostly used for detecting gait events such as heel-strike and toe-off [27].

Wearable devices can be grouped in a broad range of categories such as electrogoniometers [28], accelerometers [29], and gyroscopes [30]. For an overview on the working principle and their use in ambulatory gait analysis the reader is referred to [19,27]. Despite of all the advancements in wearable technology since 1878, some issues still persist regarding their practicality. They require precise placement and can capture only a limited amount of parameters, often requiring an array of devices for complete gait analysis [18,31]. Furthermore, a pilot study regarding the attitude of older adults to wearable devices has concluded that older persons are reluctant to use them, finding them invasive and inconvenient [32].

The last category of methods with the potential of being used ambulatory, are single camera vision-based methods. These methods use computer vision algorithms to segment the monitored person from the image background [33] and use either known body proportions [34] or have the subject wear colourized garments [35] in order to find joint locations from the segmented model. It has been concluded that the accuracy of these marker-less approaches is not yet up to par with marker-based motion capture systems [17]. Furthermore, segmenting a person from RGB data is very challenging under ambulatory conditions due to light and scene variations. A relatively young category utilizes depth data, which is invariant to illumination changes, and either use a generative [36] or a discriminative [37] model-based tracker. Generative trackers use an optimization algorithm, typically particle swarm optimization [38], to adjust the pose coefficients that minimize the quality of fit between the depth data and an a priori generated human model. Discriminative trackers use a per-pixel classification algorithm to classify each pixel to a certain body part, a human model is then regressed from this data [39]. The proprietary Microsoft SDK, a discriminative tracker, has been extensively evaluated in the context of gait analysis [40]. Discriminative trackers, however, require a vast amount of training data and the data used by Microsoft is not necessarily representative for gait analysis. For example, the Microsoft Kinect was trained with data mostly in the frontal coronal plane, while most gait disorders can be observed in the sagittal plane. Furthermore, the methods assume a static camera and conducted experiments on a treadmill, which is not representative for ambulatory monitoring. In this article, a proprietary generative tracker developed by Primesense [36] is placed on a mobile platform for over-ground monitoring. A novel method is presented for regressing spatiotemporal gait parameters from the tracked data using only the relative position of the two ankle joints. Furthermore, an implementation of a Kalman filter is presented for improving the accuracy. This approach was validated with a Vicon 10 camera motion capture system. Limitations and future work are discussed for this preliminary validation.

3   Methodology

This section is organized as follows: a description of the system components are given in Sects. 3.1 and 3.2. The validation set-up and marker placement are discussed in Sect. 3.3. Next, the extraction of gait parameters is discussed in Sect. 3.4. The coordinate transformations to a static reference frame for visualizing the results are explained in Sect. 3.5. Lastly, Sect. 3.6 discusses the implementation of the Kalman filter which is used for filtering the noisy raw joint measurements.

3.1   Following the Subject

The experimental set-up consists of a Kobuki mobile platform equipped with a Microsoft Kinect Version 1 and a laptop for data processing. The Kinect was placed at an angle of 25° relative to the ground and the robot followed the person at a distance of approximately 1.3 m, which provides a complete view of a person of average height. Figure 1 gives an overview of the experimental set-up. A wheel speed controller was developed for following the test subject throughout the validation experiments. Both the distance and angle are controlled by applying a linear or rotational velocity to the robot. The linear velocity is controlled with a state feedback controller. For controlling the rotational velocity, we assume that the person is walking in approximately a straight line throughout the experiments. The controller can thus be substantially simplified by applying a rotational velocity when the relative angle is greater than 0.1 radians.

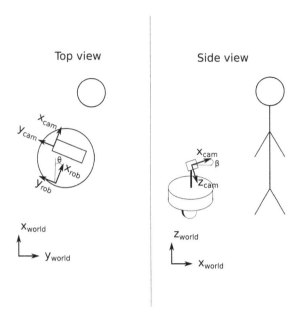

Fig. 1. Experimental set-up. Left: top view of the system. Right: side view of the system. [41].

3.2   OpenNI Tracker

To measure the 3D segmental movement of the ankle, the Microsoft Kinect and a generative propriety skeleton tracking algorithm developed by Primesense, called NITE is used [36]. An open source abstraction layer, called OpenNI [42], was used to interface the skeleton tracking middleware with the robotic operating system (ROS). The joints are presented through a transform frame [43], a ROS package that lets the user keep track of multiple coordinate frames over time, giving the 3D joint orientation relative to the moving camera frame, and the rotation through a quaternion representing the angle of the joint relative to its parent joint. For example, the rotation of the ankle joint is expressed relative to the rotation of the knee joint.

3.3   Validation Set-Up

To validate our approach, a Vicon 10 camera system that measures the 3D position of reflective markers placed on the test-subject to quantify the orientation and rotation of the foot segment, was used. Two markers were placed on each foot. Figure 2 shows the placement of the markers on the right foot and Table 1 summarizes the abbreviations of the markers.

The ankle joint center ($\vec{C}_{\text{ankle}}$) is calculated as the middle of the corresponding medial and lateral markers:

$$\vec{C}_{\text{ankle}} = 0.5 * (\vec{P}_{\text{RLA}} + \vec{P}_{\text{RMA}}) \tag{1}$$

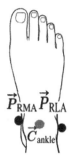

Fig. 2. Marker placement.

Table 1. Marker abbreviations.

Symbol	Description
$\vec{P}_{RMA}$	Right medial malleolus
$\vec{P}_{RLA}$	Right lateral malleolus

3.4 Extraction of Gait Parameters

Gait is described as a series of rhythmical, alternating movements of the trunk and limbs which results in the forward progression of the body. A gait cycle is defined as the time from heel contact to heel contact of the same foot. Spatial (distance) and temporal (time) parameters are used for assessing the movement of the subject. This article is an extended version of our previous work [41] in which we extract additional spatiotemporal gait parameters. In Table 2, an outline of the most commonly used spatiotemporal gait parameters is given.

Table 2. Spatio-temporal gait parameters.

Spatial parameters:	
Step length (m)	Anterior-posterior distance between successive heel contact of the opposite feet
Stride length (m)	Anterior-posterior distance between successive heel contact of the same foot
Step width (m)	Lateral distance between one heel footprint to the line of progression formed by two consecutive footprints of the opposite feet
Temporal parameters:	
Cadence (steps/min)	Amount of steps taken per minute
Single limb support (%)	Amount of time spend on a limb as a percentage of the gait cycle

A novel method was developed for deriving these spatiotemporal gait parameters similarly for both the Kinect and the Vicon data, allowing for a direct comparison. Furthermore, this method relies solely on the relative position of the two ankle joints (d_F), as opposed to the absolute position which would require accurate localization of the platform. Figure 3 shows the movement of both feet

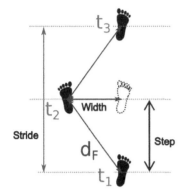

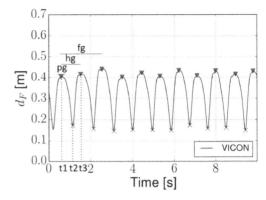

Fig. 3. Movement of both feet during half of a gait cycle.

Fig. 4. Distance between the feet as a function of time (pg = peak duration, hg = duration of half a gait cycle, fg = duration of a gait cycle).

during a typical half gait cycle and Fig. 4 shows the distance between the ankle joints of the two opposite feet as a function of time.

At time t1, the right foot is placed behind the left foot, the distance between the two ankle joints is now maximized which corresponds with the first peak at t1 in Figs. 3 and Fig. 4. Next, the swing phase of the right foot is initiated. At time t2, the right foot is in mid-swing phase, the distance between the two ankle joints is now minimized which corresponds with the first valley at t2. At time t3, the swing phase of the right foot is completed, the distance between the two ankle joints is again maximized which corresponds with the second peak at t3.

The spatial gait parameters are derived as follows. The step length of the right foot is defined as the anterior-posterior distance travelled in the duration between the valley at t2 and peak at t3. During the next (or previous) half gait cycle, the step length of the left foot can be derived. The stride length is derived as the anterior-posterior distance between t1 and t3, which is also the sum of the left and right step lengths. The step width is derived as the minimum distance between the ankle joints after offsetting the mid-flight step height.

To determine the temporal parameters, the time stamp at every consecutive peak (half of a gait cycle h_g) and every other peak (full gait cycle f_g) is extracted. The duration of half a gait cycle, which is the time for one step, can be converted to the cadence (C_g) as follows [41]:

$$C_g = \frac{60}{h_g} \tag{2}$$

Because there is no way to differentiate between heel-strike and toe-off with the OpenNI data, as opposed to an anatomically correct model, deriving the single limb support is slightly less intuitive. The time a person spends on a single limb can be derived as the time it takes to complete half of a gait cycle (h_g) minus the double stance time, which is the time a person spends on both limbs during half of a gait cycle. The double stance time can be derived as the duration of a peak, p_g in Fig. 4. To conclude, single limb support (SLS) can thus be derived as the duration of half a gait cycle (h_g) minus the duration of the double stance time (p_g), expressed as a percentage of the entire gait cycle (f_g):

$$SLS = (h_g - p_g) * \frac{100}{f_g} \tag{3}$$

3.5   Coordinate Transformations

Since the aforementioned method for extracting gait parameters relies solely on relative distances between joints, a transformation to a static frame is not necessary. However, this transformation allows for better visualization. As can be observed in Fig. 1, the first step is to compensate the angle β at which the camera is mounted relative to the floor. Next, the movement of the robot is transformed to a fixed reference frame, the starting location. The translation and rotation θ of the robot relative to the starting location is derived from the internal encoders, which are published as a transform frame similar to the joint locations by the OpenNI tracker. The joints in the world frame are thus obtained by [41]:

$$P_{world} = T_{R,rob} T_{T,rob} T_{cam} P_{cam}$$

$$T_{cam} = \begin{bmatrix} \cos\beta & 0 & \sin\beta & 0 \\ 0 & 1 & 0 & 0 \\ -\sin\beta & 0 & \cos\beta & 0 \\ 0 & 0 & 0 & 1 \end{bmatrix}$$

$$T_{T,rob} = \begin{bmatrix} 1 & 0 & 0 & x_{rob} \\ 0 & 1 & 0 & y_{rob} \\ 0 & 0 & 1 & z_{rob} \\ 0 & 0 & 0 & 1 \end{bmatrix} \tag{4}$$

$$T_{R,rob} = \begin{bmatrix} \cos\theta & -\sin\theta & 0 & 0 \\ \sin\theta & \cos\theta & 0 & 0 \\ 0 & 0 & 1 & 0 \\ 0 & 0 & 0 & 1 \end{bmatrix}$$

Where P_{world} is the joint position in the world frame, T_{cam} is the camera rotation matrix, $T_{T,rob}$ is the robot translation matrix, $T_{R,rob}$ is the robot rotation matrix, and P_{cam} is the joint position in the camera frame.

3.6   Kalman Filter

Due to tracking discontinuities prevalent in the OpenNI tracker, the raw joint positions are subject to noise, resulting in poor detection of the gait parameters. Better performance can be achieved by pre-processing the joint measurements before calculating the gait parameters. To achieve this a Kalman filter was implemented. The algorithm works according to a two step process. In the first step, a prediction of the next state is made based on a model of the system's dynamics.

This step is also called the prediction step. In the second step, a measurement is compared to a model that predicts the measurements based on the predicted state. The difference between the predicted and real measurement is weighed with the predicted state to obtain the new state estimate. Mathematically, this is expressed as [44]:

$$\hat{q}_{n|n-1} = F_n \tilde{q}_{n-1|n-1} + B_n u_n$$
$$\hat{P}_{n|n-1} = F_n \tilde{P}_{n-1|n-1} F_n^T + Q_n$$
$$\nu_n = z_n - H_n \hat{q}_{n|n-1}$$
$$K_n = \hat{P}_{n|n-1} H_n^T \left(H_n \hat{P}_{n|n-1} H_n^T + R_n \right)^{-1} \tag{5}$$
$$\tilde{q}_{n|n} = \hat{q}_{n|n-1} + K_n \nu_n$$
$$\tilde{P}_{n|n} = (I - K_n H_n) \hat{P}_{n|n-1}$$

Where q is the state vector, F is the state transition matrix, B is the control input matrix, u is the control vector, P is the covariance matrix, Q is the process noise covariance matrix, ν is the innovation, z is a measurement, K is the Kalman gain, H is the state observation matrix, R is the measurement noise covariance matrix and I is the identity matrix. Boldface symbols are used to represent matrix quantities (e.g., F). A tilde symbol is used for estimated quantities (e.g., $\tilde{q}_n$), and a hat symbol is used for predicted quantities (e.g., $\hat{y}_n$). Subscripts n, and $n-1$ are used to denote timesteps.

It can be observed that the new state is conditional only on the measurements obtained before and at the time step of the update. The Kalman filter can thus be used for near real-time gait analysis. In our case the goal is simply to smooth the data. Therefore: $F_n = 1$, $H_n = 1$, $B_n = 0$ and $u_n = 0$. The result can be compared to a moving average filter in which the window size depends on the weighted function of the process noise and the noise affecting the sensor measurements. Only knowledge of the weight of the process noise and the weight of the measurement noise must thus still be derived.

4   Results

A healthy, twenty-year-old male was used as a test subject for conducting four experiments. For each experiment, the mobile robot followed the subject from a distance of approximately 1.3 m and recorded his movement from the coronal plane. During each experiment, three gait cycles could be recorded before the subject moved out of the motion capture system's field of view. One dataset was chosen to determine the optimal Kalman filter parameters. This dataset was therefore not included in the validation results. Spatiotemporal gait parameters were extracted from the Kinect and Vicon measurements using the procedure outlined in Sect. 3.4. The Kinect measurements (J_i') are assessed in terms of mean absolute error (MAE) and mean absolute percentage error ($MAPE$) with respect to the Vicon measurements (J_i) that are considered as the 'golden standard'. The correlation between the two continuous measurement methods was assessed with the Pearson correlation coefficient (PCC). The Pearson correlation coefficient was calculated on the Euclidean distance between the two ankle joints, before calculating the gait parameters. In this section, the results of the raw and filtered measurements will be discussed.

$$MAE = \frac{1}{n} \sum_{i=1}^{n} |J_i - J_i'| \tag{6}$$

$$MAPE = \frac{100\%}{n} \sum_{i=1}^{n} \left| \frac{J_i - J_i'}{J_i} \right| \tag{7}$$

4.1   Raw Measurements

Figure 5 shows the Euclidean distance between the two ankle joints of one experiment. Table 3 summarizes the mean error and standard deviation of all the spatiotemporal gait parameters.

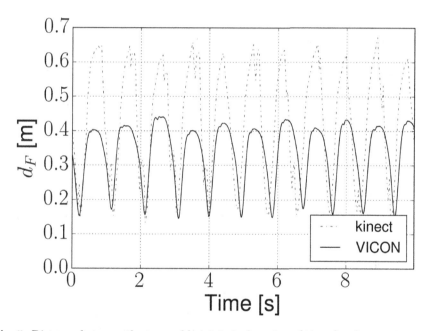

Fig. 5. Distance between the two ankle joints in function of time for the raw measurements (PCC = 0.73).

It can be observed in Fig. 5 that the OpenNI tracker consistently overestimates the maximum distance between the two ankle joints, while the minimum distance is measured accurately. Despite this overestimation, both measurement methods are highly correlated (PCC = 0.73). In Table 3 it can be observed that

Table 3. Assessment of the spatio-temporal gait parameters for the raw measurements (σ = standard deviation).

Spatial parameters	MAE $\pm\ \sigma$	MAPE (%) $\pm\ \sigma$
Step length left (m)	0.227 $\pm$ 0.030	57.8 $\pm$ 8.64
Step length right (m)	0.203 $\pm$ 0.058	52.7 $\pm$ 15.1
Stride length (m)	0.430 $\pm$ 0.064	55.1 $\pm$ 8.07
Step width (m)	0.017 $\pm$ 0.015	12.14 $\pm$ 10.6
Temporal parameters	MAE $\pm\ \sigma$	MAPE (%) $\pm\ \sigma$
Cadence (steps/min)	0.946 $\pm$ 0.194	2.68 $\pm$ 0.502
Single limb support (%)	3.40 $\pm$ 2.41	9.37 $\pm$ 7.05

the Kinect measurements show validity for the temporal parameters, but only validity for one spatial parameter. More specifically, the stride and step lengths show poor validity due to the continuous overestimation of the distance between the two ankle joints, while the step width is measured accurately. Since the NITE middleware is closed source, this phenomenon is difficult to assess. Considering the step width, measured mid-swing phase is accurate, the overestimation occurs solely near completion of a step. A likely explanation is that near the end of the swing phase it is more difficult to distinguish between the two ankle joints, which may be caused by the robot not following the person entirely straight or by the decreased depth accuracy at longer range. The tracker may then instead track a nearby body part, such as the knee. To conclude, the error on the stride and step lengths is too large to be suitable for clinical applications.

4.2   Kalman Filter

The raw data has a significant degree of noise and showed poor validity for some parameters. In order to improve performance, a Kalman filter was implemented. The filtering is carried out on the raw joint positions in the world frame before calculating the Euclidean distance between the ankle joints. The process noise and measurement noise are therefore expressed in metres. One dataset was selected to obtain the process noise and measurement noise. Through trial and error, we determined that a process noise of 0.0003 m and measurement noise of 0.03 m provide satisfactory results on this calibration dataset. Figure 6 shows the Euclidean distance between the ankle joints of one experiment after filtering the joint measurements. Table 4 summarizes the mean error and standard deviation of all the spatiotemporal gait parameters.

Table 4. Assessment of the spatio-temporal gait parameters for the filtered measurements (σ = standard deviation).

Spatial parameters	MAE $\pm\,\sigma$	MAPE (%) $\pm\,\sigma$
Step length left (m)	0.035 $\pm$ 0.096	9.67 $\pm$ 9.61
Step length right (m)	0.044 $\pm$ 0.042	10.9 $\pm$ 10.2
Stride length (m)	0.055 $\pm$ 0.035	7.14 $\pm$ 4.50
Step width (m)	0.017 $\pm$ 0.013	11.6 $\pm$ 8.34
Temporal parameters	MAE $\pm\,\sigma$	MAPE (%) $\pm\,\sigma$
Cadence (steps/min)	0.933 $\pm$ 0.441	2.62 $\pm$ 1.13
Single limb support (%)	2.54 $\pm$ 1.96	7.32 $\pm$ 5.70

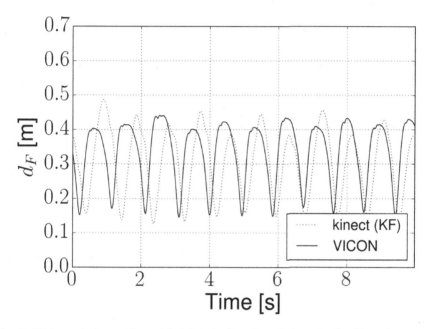

Fig. 6. Distance between the ankle joints in function of time for the filtered measurements (PCC = 0.26).

It can be observed that the accuracy has improved significantly on most parameters. The correlation between both measurement methods is, however, significantly worse (PCC = 0.26). This phenomenon is to be expected since the Kalman filter introduces a small delay. However, it is not necessary for the validation that the Kinect and the Vicon measurements are exactly time synchronized, as long as the same steps are measured.

5   Discussion

Ambulatory gait analysis methods, such as wearable devices and pressure sensors, are usually limited to very few gait parameters, thus requiring an array of sensors [18,31]. Furthermore, they are often considered inconvenient by older persons to use in daily clinical practice [32]. In this article, we presented a single camera vision-based method for unobtrusive ambulatory monitoring of a person's gait by using a mobile platform. Despite moving while tracking, similar results are achieved as static single camera set-ups. For example, Baldewijns et al. conclude a similar mean absolute error of $\pm$ 5 cm on the measurement of the stride length [45]. These results must, however, be evaluated with caution. When implementing the Kalman filter in its most basic form whereby the state transition model is an identity matrix with some added noise, as is done in this article, the filter works similar to a moving average filter. Thus, the offset between the OpenNI tracker measurements and the Vicon measurements artificially decreases. The tracker may measure one foot more accurately than the other due to self-occlusion. Artificially decreasing the offset in this situation may result in wrong assessment of the patients gait. Also, comfortable gait speed ranges from 1.3 m/s for women in their seventies to 1.5 m/s for men in their forties [46], while the mobile platform had a maximum speed of approximately 0.7 m/s. Furthermore, while the mean absolute error and mean absolute percentage error give us a preliminary idea of the validity of our method, it tells us little about the repeatability and reproducibility. This can be achieved by more thorough statistical analysis by using, for example, Bland-Altman plots [47]. These aforementioned limitations conclude that more validation experiments, with a varied patient population and a thorough statistical analysis are a necessity.

The advantage of a Kalman filter, opposed to a moving average filter, is that it can allow more complex linear models. Human motion is, however, highly nonlinear. Better results can be achieved with a non-linear variation of the Kalman filter, such as the extended or unscented Kalman filter [48], with complex human motion models.

Key gait events that are necessary for defining the gait cycle, such as heel-strike and toe-off, are typically derived from the kinematics using [26]. This method calculates heel-strike and toe-off based on the relative difference between the x-coordinate (direction of ambulation) of the heel/toe marker and the sacral marker. The OpenNI tracker, however, has no definition for the toe, this method can therefore not be used for this approach. These events could be seen on the width of the peaks, but this method likely introduces an error. Also, there is no clear anatomical meaning to the way the OpenNI tracker defines each segment. For example, there is no foot segment, as opposed to the conventional gait model [49], it is thus impossible to calculate the kinematics of the ankle (dorsiflexion and plantar flexion), limiting future extension towards kinematic parameters. A tracker that is specifically designed for the task, with an anatomically correct model, may provide a solution for these limitations.

6 Conclusion

A cost-effective method for ambulatory monitoring was presented and preliminarily validated. The Microsoft Kinect measurements are assessed in terms of mean absolute error and mean absolute percentage error with respect to the Vicon measurements. The two measurement methods are highly correlated, however, the OpenNI tracker consistently overestimates the distance between the two ankle joints. This results in poor validity for measuring step length and stride length. A Kalman filter was implemented to reduce this continuous offset. After filtering, the mean absolute error $\pm$ precision was 5.5 ± 3.5 cm for stride length, 1.7 ± 1.3 cm for step width, 0.93 ± 0.44 steps/min for cadence, and $2.5 \pm 2.0\%$ for single limb support. Whether the accuracy of this approach is sufficient for ambulatory monitoring depends on the desired accuracy of the specific task. Several limitations to this approach were discussed. In summary, the validation experiments were conducted on a single healthy person and motion was measured solely from the coronal plane, in a controlled laboratory environment. Additional studies are therefore necessary to further investigate the applicability of this method when monitoring frailer, older adults. Furthermore, several limitations were found that are inherent to the used proprietary tracker, limiting further expandability.

Acknowledgements. The authors would like to thank MALL (Movements posture & Analysis Laboratory Leuven) of the Faculty of Movement and Rehabilitation Sciences Leuven for providing the facility equipped with a VICON motion capture system in order to validate the proposed platform. Robin Amsters is an SB fellow of the Research Foundation Flanders (FWO) under grant agreement 1S57718N.

References

1. United Nations, World population ageing 2015 (ST/ESA/SER.A/390). Technical Report 1, Department of Economic and Social Affairs, Population Division (2015)
2. Nimmesgern, E., Benediktsson, I., Norstedt, I.: Clin. Transl. Sci. **10**(2), 61 (2017)
3. G.S. of the Council to Delegations, Council Conclusions (2015)
4. European Commission, Research and Innovation. Conferences and Events: Personalised Medicine Conference 2016 (2016)
5. Bemelmans, R., Gelderblom, G.J., Jonker, P., de Witte, L.: J. Am. Med. Dir. Assoc. **13**(2), 114 (2012)
6. Wada, K., Shibata, T., Saito, T., Tanie, K.: Proc. IEEE **92**(11), 1780 (2004)
7. Gaugler, J.E., Yu, F., Krichbaum, K., Wyman, J.F.: Med. Care **47**(2), 191 (2009)
8. Valkanova, V., Ebmeier, K.P.: Gait Posture **53**, 215 (2017)
9. Salarian, A., et al.: IEEE Trans Biomed. Eng. **51**(8), 1434 (2004)
10. Viswanathan, A., Sudarsky, L.: Handb. Clin. Neurol. **103**, 623 (2012)
11. Moore, S.T., Dilda, V., Hakim, B., Macdougall, H.G.: Biomed. Eng. Online **10**, 82 (2011)
12. Fahn, S.: Recent Developments in Parkinson's Disease, vol. 2, p. 153 (1987)
13. Ijmker, T., Lamoth, C.J.C.: Gait Posture **35**(1), 126 (2012)
14. Del Din, S., Godfrey, A., Galna, B., Lord, S., Rochester, L.: J. Neuroeng. Rehabil. **13**(1), 46 (2016)

15. DeLisa, J.A.: Gait Analysis in the Science of Rehabilitation. DIANE Publishing, Darby (1998)
16. Mündermann, L., Corazza, S., Andriacchi, T.P.: J. Neuroeng. Rehabil. **3**, 6 (2006)
17. Ceseracciu, E., Sawacha, Z., Cobelli, C.: PLoS One **9**(3), e87640 (2014)
18. Muro-de-la Herran, A., García-Zapirain, B., Méndez-Zorrilla, A.: Gait analysis methods: an overview of wearable and non-wearable systems, highlighting clinical applications (2014)
19. Tao, W., Liu, T., Zheng, R., Feng, H.: Sensors **12**(2), 2255 (2012)
20. Razak, A.H.A., Zayegh, A., Begg, R.K., Wahab, Y.: Sensors **12**(7), 9884 (2012)
21. Toro, B., Nester, C., Farren, P.: Physiother. Theory Pract. **19**(3), 137 (2003)
22. Fahrenberg, J.: Ambulatory Assessment: Computer-Assisted Psychological and Psychophysiological Methods in Monitoring and Field Studies, pp. 3–20 (1996)
23. Marey, E.J.: La méthode graphique dans les sciences expérimentales et principalement en physiologie et en médecine. G. Masson (1878)
24. Hausdorff, J.M., Ladin, Z., Wei, J.Y.: J. Biomech. **28**(3), 347 (1995)
25. Jagos, H., et al.: J. Med. Eng. Technol. **41**(5), 375 (2017)
26. Zeni Jr., J.A., Richards, J.G., Higginson, J.S.: Gait Posture **27**(4), 710 (2008)
27. Rueterbories, J., Spaich, E.G., Larsen, B., Andersen, O.K.: Med. Eng. Phys. **32**(6), 545 (2010)
28. Myles, C.M., Rowe, P.J., Walker, C.R.C., Nutton, R.W.: Gait Posture **16**(1), 46 (2002)
29. Senden, R., Grimm, B., Heyligers, I.C., Savelberg, H.H.C.M., Meijer, K.: Gait Posture **30**(2), 192 (2009)
30. Aminian, K., et al.: Gait Posture **20**(1), 102 (2004)
31. Yang, C.C., Hsu, Y.L.: Sensors **10**(8), 7772 (2010)
32. Demiris, G., et al.: Med. Inform. Internet Med. **29**(2), 87 (2004)
33. Baldewijns, G., et al.: J. Ambient. Intell. Smart Environ. **8**(3), 273 (2016). https://lirias.kuleuven.be/retrieve/427059/Paper_publish.pdf [Available for KU Leuven users]
34. Goffredo, M., Carter, J.N., Nixon, M.S.: 2D markerless gait analysis. In: Vander, S.J., Verdonck, P., Nyssen, M., Haueisen, J. (eds.) 4th European Conference of the International Federation for Medical and Biological Engineering. IFMBE Proceedings, vol. 22, pp. 67–71. Springer, Heidelberg (2009). https://doi.org/10.1007/978-3-540-89208-3_18
35. Castelli, A., Paolini, G., Cereatti, A., Della Croce, U.: Comput. Math. Methods Med. **2015**, 186780 (2015)
36. PrimeSense Inc.: Prime Sensor^{TM} NITE 1.3 Algorithms notes (2010). http://pr.cs.cornell.edu/humanactivities/data/NITE.pdf. Accessed 07 June 2018
37. Shotton, J., et al.: IEEE Trans Pattern Anal. Mach. Intell. **35**(12), 2821 (2013)
38. Zhang,X., Hu, W., Maybank, S., Li, X., Zhu, M.: 2008 IEEE Conference on Computer Vision and Pattern Recognition, pp. 1–8 (2008)
39. Supancic, J.S., Rogez, G., Yang, Y., Shotton, J., Ramanan, D.: 2015 IEEE International Conference on Computer Vision (ICCV), pp. 1868–1876 (2015)
40. Springer, S., Yogev Seligmann, G.: Sensors **16**(2), 194 (2016)
41. Amsters, R., et al.: Proceedings of the 4th International Conference on Information and Communication Technologies for Ageing Well and e-Health, pp. 49–61. SCITEPRESS - Science and Technology Publications (2018)
42. OpenNI Organization: OpenNI User Guide (2010). https://github.com/OpenNI/OpenNI/blob/master/Documentation/OpenNI_UserGuide.pdf. Accessed 07 June 2018

43. Foote, T.: 2013 IEEE International Conference on Technologies for Practical Robot Applications (TePRA), Open-Source Software workshop, pp. 1–6 (2013). https://doi.org/10.1109/TePRA.2013.6556373

44. Thrun, S., Burgard, W., Fox, D.: Probabilistic Robotics (Intelligent Robotics and Autonomous Agents). The MIT Press, Cambridge (2005)

45. Baldewijns, G., Verheyden, G., Vanrumste, B., Croonenborghs, T.: Proceedings Conference of IEEE Engineering in Medicine and Biology Society, p. 5920 (2014)

46. Bohannon, R.W.: Age Ageing **26**(1), 15 (1997)

47. Altman, D.G., Bland, J.M.: J. R. Stat. Society. Ser. D (Stat.) **32**(3), 307 (1983)

48. Julier, S.J., Uhlmann, J.K.: Signal Processing, Sensor Fusion, and Target Recognition VI, vol. 3068, pp. 182–194. International Society for Optics and Photonics (1997)

49. Charalambous, C.P.: Measurement of lower extremity kinematics during level walking. In: Banaszkiewicz, P.A., Kader, D.F. (eds.) Classic Papers Orthopaedics, pp. 397–398. Springer, London (2014). https://doi.org/10.1007/978-1-4471-5451-8_100

Studying the Acceptance of a Digital Diabetes Diaries

André Calero Valdez[✉] and Martina Ziefle

Human-Computer Interaction Center, RWTH Aachen University,
Campus-Boulevard 57, Aachen, Germany
{calero-valdez,ziefle}@comm.rwth-aachen.de

Abstract. The incidence of diabetes has increased dramatically in recent years and this trend is expected to continue. It is essential for the therapy of diabetes that patients keep a diary. However, diary keeping is often incomplete and digitally supported diaries are poorly accepted by older patients. With the help of focus groups, we collected requirements for a digital diabetes diary and implemented them using a LiveScribe pen. This digitally augmented pen allows you to keep the diary traditionally on paper and still offer digital support. By digitizing an already known process, our solution achieves a high level of acceptance even among older people. The evaluation was carried out with the help of the TAM model and was used to quantify the effects of user factors. Typical predictors of acceptance do not work in our model, which we see as an indication that our pen is not perceived as technology in the classical sense.

Keywords: Usability testing · Novel interaction paradigms ·
Pen computing · User centered design ·
Empirical studies in interaction design

1 Introduction

The Internet of Things [1] and the ubiquitous availability of computing power [2] makes it possible for any device to be connected to the Internet and to send and receive data. Can this change in the technology landscape lead to fewer barriers for people using medical technology [3]?

Although many theories assume that the usefulness of a device determines its acceptance [4], it must be taken into account that acceptance is neither a static nor a very predictable concept. This applies in particular to the acceptance of medical technology, as a disease changes the patient over time—similar to aging. If medical technology is very noticeable, this can represent a further barrier for the user. This applies in particular to users who already feel dependent on modern technology and deliberately refuse to use it. Nevertheless, many users use ICT every day when they enter an elevator, when they drive, when they use their phones. The visibility of technology has an impact on acceptance. And

© Springer Nature Switzerland AG 2019
P. D. Bamidis et al. (Eds.): ICT4AWE 2018, CCIS 982, pp. 142–166, 2019.
https://doi.org/10.1007/978-3-030-15736-4_8

acceptance of ubiquitous medical device support increases when the technology is integrated in a patient's trusted environment [5]. Benefits and drawbacks of such solutions must naturally be evaluated [6].

In this article we describe an approach for a Digital Diabetes Diary, which hides the technology from the user in the background and integrates the technology into existing behavioural patterns. The diary hides the assistance functions in the pen with which the entries in the diary are maintained. It is an extension of previous work and provides a deeper look into the technological details of the prototype [7].

1.1 Demographic Change and Diabetes

The demography in Western nations changes. Life expectancy increases, birth rates decrease, the amount of people with an age of 60 and older will quadruple by the year 2050 [8]. According to the [9] Germany will have at least 22 million seniors older than 65 years in 2060. With increased life expectancy comes increased wealth, technological progress, and a sedentary lifestyle [10]. The problem with an aging [11] and sedentary [12] population is that the prevalence of illnesses like diabetes increases.

1.2 Obstacles in Diabetes Therapy

If diabetes is not or only poorly treated, it causes a variety of damage to the organs (e.g. neurological, cardiological, etc.). This results in extremely high treatment costs compared to patients whose treatment is well adjusted [13].

The biggest challenge in diabetes therapy consists in adapting the therapy to the patient and then adhering to it [13,14]. In order to address the individual aspects of each patients illness, patients are required to keep a diabetes diary. In this diary vital parameters such as blood glucose levels are recorded along with insulin dosages, activity data, and food intake. The doctor must now understand the idiosyncratic reactions of the patients body to medication and lifestyle and adjust therapy accordingly.

Quality of therapy is highly dependent on the quality of the diary keeping [11]. Users often refrain from keeping their diary in a precise fashion, but often fill their diary at the end of the day from memory [15]. It is necessary for a diabetic to calculate the insulin doses using cross-multiplication, as the dosage is both dependent on current glucose levels and a correctional factor that is individually established for different times of the day. Also, a persisting diabetes can also lead to cognitive deficits [16,17], which in turn hampers therapy.

2   Related Work

In the following we review the literature on digital diabetes diaries and management applications. From the literature we see different forms of application and input methods. Generally electronic and paper based diaries have been investigated with differing results. We then introduce the LiveScribe Echo Pen, which was used in an approach to combine the best of both worlds—a digital pen paper-based diabetes diary, that provides a multitude of the features that typical electronic diaries provide.

2.1   Diabetes Management

Several system have been proposed to improve diabetes care. Early approaches like DEMS [18,19] have tried to build a PDA based diabetes management program, that uses a client-server architecture in order store data on the web. DEMS allows that the patient keeps track of his diet, exercise, blood sugar levels, and his medication. DEMS was also assessed for its usability.

As early as 2003 Kerkenbush conducted a study on the efficacy of PDA-based diabetes diaries against paper-based diabetes diaries. Kerkenbush and Lasome [20] identified the importance of PDA based solutions for diabetes care. They identified the importance of systematic and regular tracking in a diabetes diary for patients health as well as the need to teach potential users how to use a PDA based diary system.

The use of PDA based diabetes diaries is in particularly interesting as Stone et al. [15] found a high unwillingness to paper diaries in many diabetes patients. This is not necessarily caused by a lack of therapy adherence but might have been caused by simple forgetting. An electronic device could have a reminder function, leading to a possible increase in diary keeping.

Broderick and Stone [21] argue though, that comparability in regard to the device type is not yet possible. Reasons for compliance rates are not assessable through the conducted studies and could be conflicted by errors of self-reporting, motivation, and lack of actual medical compliance analysis.

Nonetheless, Forjuoh et al. [22] investigated the medical impact of using PDA based diaries between high and low usage of the PDA software "Diabetes Pilot". Over a course of six months high usage resulted in an significantly better increase in vital parameters than in low usage users. Still both groups showed improved of their vital parameters.

Duke et al. [23] developed the Intelligent Diabetes Assistant (IDA). IDA uses machine learning algorithms to improve therapy by measuring lifestyle, nutrition and glucose levels. The measurements are instantly shared with a physician to allow shorter feedback loops on the diary evaluation. A similar solution has been developed by Tani et al. [24], which was also evaluated positively.

According to [25] technological assistance in diabetes therapy will increase in importance in particular in conjunction with closed-loop therapies. New Technologies will emerge and play a bigger role in keeping patients healthy.

Burke et al. [26] investigated the differences in monitoring food intake on a PDA after training hemodialysis and weight-loss patients in using a digital food diary. They found a higher loss of weight and higher self-monitoring adherence in users of a PDA based diary than users of paper-based diaries [27]. If daily feedback was given through the PDA improvements were even larger.

When looking at PDAs [28] and mobile phones [29] acceptance of these devices might depend on prior experience and in particular be important when the users are part of the target demographic—elderly users.

In a time when the technical challenges are no longer the largest barriers, it becomes important the regard the users emotive, hedonic [30] and cultural needs [31], especially when developing medical technology. Users might have a preference of using paper over PDAs or mobile phones for sheer haptic reasons [32]. When specifically looking at diabetes devices age shows a particular negative influence on usage performance [33]. Additionally the screen size of the device increases usability in particular for older users [34,35]. Since some users are not familiar with the hierarchical menu structures of mobile phones or PDAs, other forms of navigation through a device should be considered [34]. This is particularly the case in mobile devices, where screen real-estate is scarce and can not be using excessively for user guidance.

2.2   Anoto-Paper

Pen-based information input dates back to the mid 1990ies, when the Apple Newton was devised. Primary research [36] dealt with how a PDA that used pen-based input could be leveraged to assist engineers. Back then intelligence lay in the PDA and not in the pen. Pettersson et al. [37] filed a patent in 2005 describing an approach to map a position on a piece of printed paper to an absolute virtual coordinate using an infrared camera. The camera is mounted into a pen allowing the pen to "know" where it is writing, when the paper has a specific pattern printed onto it (see Fig. 1).

The pattern assumes a virtual grid on paper and uses the offset of printed dots from this grid to code the position of the paper. The pattern uses a $1.8 \times 1.8 \,\mathrm{mm}$ grid making it barely visible to the human eye. The dots only have a diameter of about $60 - 100 \,\mu\mathrm{m}$. 6×6 dots encode four bits are used to code a coordinate allowing to encode for 4^{6*6} bits of information per position. This allows to uniquely address $4.6 * 10^7$ km^2 of paper [38][1].

2.3   Livescribe Echo

The Anoto Pattern has been licensed to multiple companies among them *Livescribe*, who produces three different variations of their *Echo* pen, differing mostly in regard to memory size. This pen can be used for a multitude of applications [39]. Traditional applications are recording audio-data along with written notes (e.g. in lectures). But the audio input/output interface along with absolute position tracking of the pen's tip, allows for more complex interactions patterns.

Livescribe was the only licensee that offered an SDK that allowed user-development of pen-based applications that run on the pen independently. The

---

[1] This equals to approx. 1% of the earths surface.

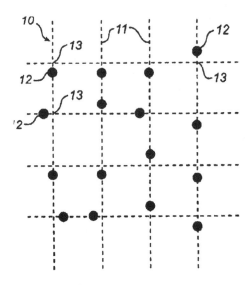

Fig. 1. The ANOTO pattern. Dashed lines are virtual lines, not printed. Dots-offsets encode absolute position. Image taken from [37].

Livescribe Echo enabled for programmable user interaction when the user writes on Anoto-Paper.[2]

All versions of the *Livescribe Echo* are based on an ARM9 processor. The pen is larger (158×19 mm) and heavier (36 g) than an average pen. Data transfer happens using a micro-USB connector. The pen also has a 96×18 pixel OLED-Display, an integrated microphone and integrated loudspeaker. It also has a headphone jack, which further allows recording of stereo-data.

The *Livescribe Platform SDK* is available in Version 1.5 and Livescribe Desktop in Version 0.7. The *Livescribe Echo* also supports the *Livescribe Java API*.

Applications built for the *Livescribe Echo* are called *Penlets*. *Penlets* have access to the on-board optical character recognition library and can therefore recognize letters and numbers that are written with the pen.

2.4   Technology Acceptance

Since actual usage of devices depends largely on user acceptance it is necessary to incorporate acceptance modeling in the development process of such a device. For our case we have chosen to rely on the Technology Acceptance Model (TAM) by Davis [40]. TAM based the intention to use a system on two explaining variables. The perceived ease of use (PEU) and perceived usefulness (PU) determine largely the behavioral intention.

---

[2] Unfortunately, Livescribe changes this feature in the meantime, and the SDK is currently unavailable.

Other models such as UTAUT [41], TAM2 [42] and TAM3 [43] were also considered but are not used due to the amount of factors that they introduce to the method. The TAM model has successfully been used to model the acceptance of medical technology in a health care setting [42].

3 Requirement Analysis

In order to develop a Livescribe-based diabetes-management-assistant that is both usable and accepted the user must be taken into account. To get insights into the life of a diabetic a focus group was conducted, the results of which are presented next.

3.1 Focus Group Results

The focus group was conducted in order to get first insights into using a mobile device for diabetics. In order to guarantee focus group success a list of core questions was initially established, which were then given to the participants. The questions were picked with five topics in mind.

The first topic is "diabetes in general" and questions were selected with special focus on therapy and diabetes management. The second topic is "mobile devices". The questions regarding this topic were selected to understand the impact of the level of technology expertise in using medical technology (i.e. mobile devices for diabetics). Special focus was put on the features of the used devices and their acceptance. The third topic is "diabetes diaries". Questions for this topic were chosen to improve understanding of how potential users keep their diary. The last two topics are usage motives and barriers. Questions for these topics were picked to assess future hurdles to prevent when implementing a device.

Five participants contributed to this setting and shared the following demographic information:

1. Type 1 diabetic, male 26 years, student of Computer Science, athlete
2. Type 1 diabetic, female, 14 years, pupil (accompanied by her mother)
3. Type 1 diabetic, female, 42 years, civil servant, Insulin-pump
4. Type 2 diabetic, male, 46 years, university degree in Mathematics
5. Type 2 diabetic, male, 63 years, retiree,

Results. In the focus group five participants were asked to elaborate on the experience with diabetes, mobile devices, diabetes management and possible motives and barriers for using a diabetes management assistant. The participants were selected from a pro-active group of diabetics (i.e. visitors of a diabetes congress), they were self-selected, and had no known secondary disorders. They were mostly well-educated and all on insulin therapy.

The most important findings that would need consideration from this focus group are (in order of occurrence):

1. Diabetes in general
   (a) Diabetes strongly influences the daily routine.
   (b) Physical activity needs special attention.
   (c) Willingness to adhere is high, but mood dependent.
   (d) Domain knowledge of diabetes is high, but varies with severity of the disease.
   (e) Informedness varies with understanding of diabetes.
   (f) Different parameters are known differently well depending on (perceived) domain knowledge.
   (g) Important parameters are blood glucose level, HbA_1c, body-fat percentage & blood pressure.
2. Mobile devices
   (a) Insulin pumps are perceived as very helpful, but sometimes as foreign.
   (b) General satisfaction with devices is high.
   (c) Advanced functions are not used.
3. Diabetes diaries
   (a) Paper-based diary keeping is common but perceived as cumbersome.
   (b) Shortcuts are used to simplify logging.
4. Motives and barriers
   (a) Therapy is cumbersome and device implementation a necessity.
   (b) Operating expense (i.e. time) must be minimal.
   (c) Some people prefer paper-based diaries over digital ones.
   (d) Data safety is important.
   (e) Low level of perceived usefulness might be a barrier.
   (f) Benefits for health are imaginable if the device integrates well into the daily routine.
   (g) Insulin-dosing calculation would be a helpful feature.
   (h) Deal-breakers are bad usability and public visibility.
   (i) Mobile phone integration is only attractive for some users.

4   An Interactive Anoto-Paper Based Diabetes Diary

From the requirements gathered, we conceptualized a diabetes diary using the *Livescribe Echo* digital pen. The idea behind the software named *Diabetto* was to let users keep their paper-based diaries but offer interactive support using the *Livescribe Echo*. This pen uses an infrared-camera to detect what is being written with the pen and has a microphone and loudspeaker included. Both can be used from software on the pen. Usage feels like using a normal pen on regular paper, but with digital support.

All versions of the *Livescribe Echo* are based on an ARM9 processor. The pen is larger ($158 \times 19\,mm$) and heavier ($36\,g$) than an average pen. Data transfer happens using a micro-USB connector. The pen also has a 96×18 pixel OLED-Display, an integrated microphone and integrated loudspeaker. It also has a headphone jack, which further allows recording of stereo-data.

The software Diabetto does not focus on the evaluation of generic diabetes diary keeping, but on assisting the user by verbal feedback on diary entries.

Furthermore it should allow self-defined shortcuts the simplify diary keeping in order to reduce barriers. The following section introduces how the Diabetto software was developed, which is then evaluated in the next section.

4.1   Diabetto – A Digital Pen Based Diabetes Diary

The first essential part of Diabetto is the paper-based diary. The diary consists of three parts. The first part is the actual diary pages that the users uses to log his diary entries. The second part is a set of pages that contain a database of food items that the user can modify as a shortcut to regularly consumed meals. The last part is a set of general abbreviations that allows the user to record and input with a self-defined abbreviation.

The Diary Pages. The first part is the actual diary (see Fig. 2). The diary itself consists of lined paged that are empty. Each page refers to a certain day. Users can write on these lines indicating what they have done on a particular day.

When a line starts with a *time-information* (e.g. 9:00) the diary assumes this to be the time of the entry (used when logging forgotten information). When no time is given the current system time is used as the time of entry. Time-information is recognized by a regular expression detecting any four or five set of numerical characters with a colon in between.

Blood glucose readings are detected, when a line ends with the characters "bs". The pen then tries to recognize the number before these characters and interprets them and gives advice accordingly. When the numbers are on the low end of health blood glucose levels an auditory warning is issued:"Warning, your glucose levels are low. Please verify your measurement or react to this state." When levels were too high an analogous warning was issued. This message also included a suggestion of how much insulin to administer in order to reduce the amount of blood glucose level to a healthy level. In the case of normal measurements a confirmatory message containing the numerical value written in the diary was played.

Whenever the two characters "BU" are found after numerical characters a *food consumption* entry is assumed. The amount of BU-units is played as auditory feedback and then recorded.

Insulin dosages were recognized when the characters "IU" were found after numerical characters. Auditory feedback on the amount of administered international units of insulin was played.

When a word is written that ends with a question mark, the pen looks into his *nutrition facts* or *abbreviation database*. If an entry in the nutrition facts exists, the amount of BU-units is reported to the user using audio feedback. If the same word is written with a dot at the end, the BU-units are recorded as a diary entry. Found abbreviations are "unfolded" and the reinterpreted.

The rest of the line, which is not interpreted, is used as a *commentary* to the respective diary entry.

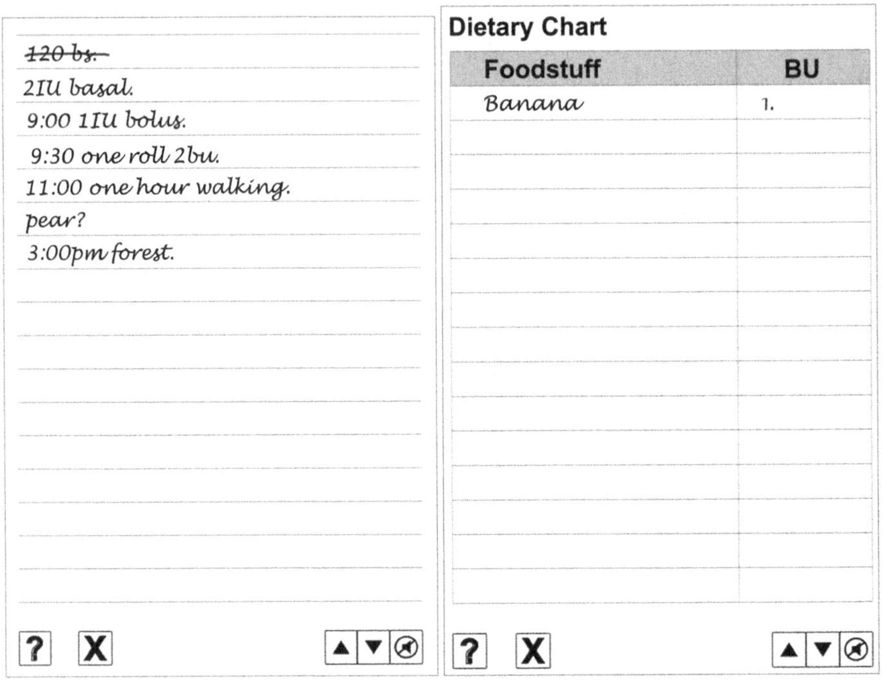

Fig. 2. A sample diary page (left). The diary page contains a list of entries, one per line. Entries that are striked-through are deleted entries. Entries that have no time are recorded using the system time. Example page of the Diabetto diary showing a nutrition facts sheet (right). A user may write food items he consumes often in the left column and its BU-units in the right column. Figure from [7].

If no interpretable data is contained in a single row, the entry is recorded as an *activity* (e.g. "one hour walking").

Entries can be *deleted* either by striking them through or by clicking the X-button on the bottom of the page immediately after input.

Furthermore every page has a *help* button (showing a "?") that starts a short audio-tutorial to the pen, as well as three buttons to *adjust the volume* of the pen (i.e. volume up/down/mute).

The Nutrition Facts Pages. The second part of the diary contains a table with columns (see Fig. 2). The left column is used to enter the name of a meal or a food item that should be stored in the diary. The right column (in the same row) takes the amount of BU-units that are associated with this entry. These entries can be used in the diary as a shortcut. Furthermore deletion of entries is possible by striking them through.

The Abbreviations Pages. The third and last part of the diary is very similar to the second part. It also has two columns. The left column takes the abbreviation, while the right column takes the expanded full text. Whenever a user writes a word from the left column of the abbreviations pages the text of right column of the same row is virtually inserted and interpreted. This allows for complex abbreviations like "9:00 Breakfast, 2 cheese rolls, 6BU." that may occur regularly in a users life.

4.2   The Applications

Two applications are part of Diabetto. The first application is the penlet that runs within the pen to provide the functionality of the diary. Since any of the features that were described in the previous section are actually a functionality of the pen and not the paper, no detailed further information about the penlet application is necessary. This already indicates that the pen itself is not considered as the interface, but the paper is, although technically the opposite applies. The application automatically starts, when the pen is used on Diabetto-diary paper. The second application is desktop-application to synchronize data. This application is not part of our evaluation here.

5   Questions Addressed

Classical technology acceptance using a TAM model requires to assess the usefulness and ease of use of a technology to estimate the behavioral intention to use the technology. In our case we wanted further information to be available for analysis.

We were interested in finding out whether the auditory-feedback and the writing-based input were usable and helpful to the patients. We assumed that the integration into the already known process of keeping a paper-based diary would be easier than teaching a PDA or mobile phone application. Additionally we were interested in seeing how age, expertise, domain knowledge, and computer self-efficacy influenced the evaluation of the device, as previous studies had shown a strong influence of these factors [33,35] in PDA based devices. In particular the effectiveness of use has shown to be good predictor of perceived ease of use in previous exploratory studies [33]. Under the assumption that a pen might be less likely seen as a technological device, influences off effectiveness during use could differ from previous studies.

6   Experimental Evaluation

In order to understand, whether possible users would accept a digital paper-based diary and how well they could use such a device, a user study was conducted. Focus of the study was to let users use the pen in a scenario-based task, assess their performance and furthermore assess their acceptance of the device.

6.1   Method

The experiments were conducted at the RWTH Aachen in a laboratory environment. Additional experiments were conducted at the office of Dr. Lätzsch in Aachen in order to remove some effect of the self-selection that occurs when participants have to travel to the experimental destination. Participants were directly contacted in the physician's office or for the control group taken from the immediate social network of the author.

6.2   Experimental Procedure

The experiment was conducted in several steps. First participants were informed about the experiment and that their data was being recorded. In order to measure performance, videos of the experiments were also recorded. The participant was informed that the interaction would be recorded on video, not exposing the face (only the diary and the hand were in frame). Then participants had to answer a questionnaire.

In order to get accustomed to the digital pen, first four tasks were instructed, in which the participant would also receive assistance from the experimenter. These tasks could also be repeated as often as desired. Once a participant stated that he understood the concept behind the digital pen, participants were instructed to perform three performance tasks. After finishing the task sets, a post-experimental questionnaire had to be answered. After this last questionnaire participants were instructed about how they could contact the experimenter in case they wanted any of the data deleted at any time afterwards.

6.3   The Questionnaire

The questionnaire was separated in two parts. Participants were asked demographic data such as age, gender and work. Furthermore handedness was assessed because handedness could influence accuracy of the text recognition.

Additionally health status was assessed. This means type of diabetes, diabetes duration and type of therapy were assessed. Technical expertise was assessed with both household and expertise in computerized technology (ECT) as well as expertise in health technology (EHT). For descriptive purposes coping scales and domain knowledge scales were assessed (i.e. DP, DCI, TDC, IFG, IFO).

Lastly the computer self-efficacy (CSE) [44] and behavioral intention to use the diary were assessed. Computer self-efficacy was measured using eight items, while behavioral intention was measured using three items.

6.4   The Task Set

In order to assure equal conditions between participants a fixed task set was designed, which included all features of the Diabetto diary. Instructions were available in paper-based format (i.e. printed between the pre- and post-questionnaire). Questions to the experimenter were allowed during the first four tasks. The following four tasks were used as introductory tasks:

1. **Opening the Help Function.** Users were asked to activate the help function. This task required them to understand that they could "click" on buttons on the paper, which activates behavior of the pen. Furthermore participants were encouraged to set the audio level output to a comfortable level.
2. **Write a Simple Sentence.** Users were asked to write in a line of the diary "I am taking part in an experiment". To this entry the pen would give audio feedback: "An activity for <date of experiment> was logged". This introduced the participant to the idea that the diary recognizes input as a diary and stores the information.
3. **Log a Glucose Measurement.** Users were asked to add an entry to the diary saying that they had a blood glucose reading of 100 mg/dl. The pen would give audio feedback and comment on the healthy value of 100. This introduced participants to the idea that the diary could be used to record glucose measurements, and that the pen would comment on the value.
4. **Log Insulin Dosing.** Users were asked to log two entries of insulin dosing. This introduced the participants to how insulin dosing can be logged in Diabetto.

After completing the introductory tasks, the participant was informed that the following tasks were the actual experiment. Then the performance task sets were presented. The task set consisted of the following complex tasks:

5. **Log a Whole Day.** The user was asked to record typical measurements and doses and activities of a whole day in the diary.
6. **Usage of Nutrition Facts.** The users were asked to retrieve the BU-unit value for an already stored food item from the database. Furthermore they were asked to create their own entry and retrieve that value as well.
7. **Usage of Abbreviations.** Users were asked to create an abbreviation and use it in the diary.

After the completion of these tasks, the pen was connected to a Laptop and the Desktop application was shown, as well as a printout of the diary entries was handed to the participants.

In some cases participants strayed from doing the actual task, because the data given in the task did not coincide with their personal life. In those cases, participants were gently reminded and asked whether they could, after entering the own personal data, complete the actual task. This behavior deemed successful because participant's curiosity, how the pen behaved in their own lives was satisfied, but nonetheless all tasks were completed.

In cases were the pen did not recognize readings, and when it was obvious that recognition failure was caused by the limited dictionary provided by the prototype, participants were reminded of the prototypical nature of the experiment, and asked to retry the task using the words given in the task description. The amount of additional help was noted for additional evaluation.

6.5   Performance Measurement

In order to analyze performance video data is analyzed using a form sheet. The sheet has predefined actions that when recognized in the video recording are counted for evaluation. Approx. 14 hours of video data was analyzed for the data.

Items that are counted are the participant's security in using the device (i.e. "asks for help" and "corrects mistakes on his own") and user satisfaction (i.e. "positive mentions of the device", "negative mentions of the device", "laughter"). Additionally it is recorded whether the participant ignores visual and auditory feedback of the device.

Furthermore it is recorded when technical problems (e.g. OCR fails) occur, what participants say about the device and a general impression of the experimenter of the participant.

Timing is measured by entering the time-codec of the frame when a user clearly starts reading a task, when he starts writing, and when he finishes writing (i.e. the pen is lifted). Furthermore it is noted whether the task was effectively completed.

Time on task was calculated as the difference of finishing time codec from start time codec.

7   Hypotheses

As independent variables demography and health values were used. Age, gender and diabetes related factors were assessed. Furthermore expertise with technology and domain knowledge, as well as computer self-efficacy were assessed. As intermediary variables task performance was measures in regard to effectiveness and efficiency. Lastly as dependent variables perceived ease of use and perceived usefulness were assessed in order to assess influence on behavioral intention (see Fig. 3).

We assume that age influences computer self-efficacy negatively (H_1), similar as age should influence expertise with technology negatively (H_2). Both these factors, as shown in previous experiments, should influence the efficiency during the experiment (H_3). The effectiveness of using a diabetes diary in general should be positively influence (H_4) by either knowing more about diabetes or being more experienced in using diabetes diaries (i.e. longer diabetes duration). Efficiency and Effectiveness should both influence the perception of ease using the diary (H_5), while perceived usefulness should also depend on experience, our previous experiments have not confirmed this finding [33]. Therefore this is not a formulated hypothesis. Furthermore we expect to see a positive influence on behavioral intention using both PEU and PU (H_6).

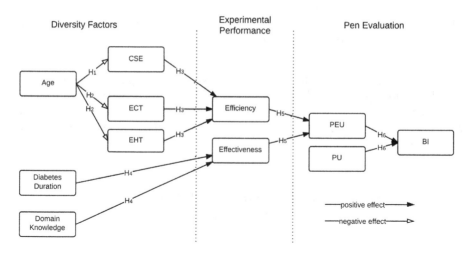

Fig. 3. Visual representation of hypotheses. Figure from [7]

8   Sample Description

A set of 27 participants took part in the study. The average age was 38 years ($SD = 15.8$, 22–73 years). Eleven participants were male (41%), and 16 were female. Eight participants were diabetics. Three persons were left-handed. Healthy participants were recruited from announcements in a local newspaper, and diabetics via the social network of diabetes patients.

The participants were split in three groups (tertial-split) according to their age. The young age group showed a mean age of 25 ($SD = 2.7$, $n = 10$), the medium age group showed a mean age of 34 years ($SD = 5.7$, $n = 10$), and the old age group showed a mean age of 62 ($SD = 5.7$, $n = 7$).

Diabetics showed a mean age of 49 years ($SD = 17.7$), while non-diabetics only showed a mean age of 33 years ($SD = 12.7$). Mann-Whitney-U testing reveals that diabetics were indeed older than non-diabetics ($U = 35.5$, $z = -2.157$, $p < .05$, $r = -.42$).

9   Results

In the following sections results are presented. Results are analyzed using bi-variate correlations, univariate analysis of variance (ANOVA) and multiple linear regression analysis.

9.1   Descriptive Results

In order to get a broad overview into the results, first descriptive statistics for the three age groups are presented. When a influence seem plausible, correlation data is also presented. First we look into perception of aging and technical expertise.

Then diabetes scales are presented. Lastly the various performance metrics, as well as a pen evaluation is presented.

Technical Expertise. Technical expertise seems to be highly and equally well distributed for the ECT and EHT scale (see Fig. 4). Only expertise with medical technology is very low for all age groups. Computer self-efficacy seems to decrease with age. Overall the sample seems to be highly tech-savvy with the typical decrease in self-efficacy with age.

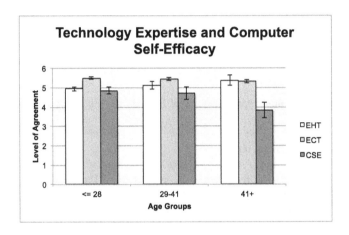

Fig. 4. Technical expertise and efficacy scale marginal means over age. EHT = Expertise with household technology, ECT = Expertise with computerized technology, CSE = Computer self-efficacy. Error bars denote standard error. Figure from [7].

Correlation analysis confirms that age correlates significantly with computer self-efficacy (CSE). ($r = .-457$, $p < .05$). Interestingly the seemingly equal technology expertise with computerized technology (ECT) correlates highly significantly with the CSE ($r = .577$, $p < .01$).

Diabetes: Coping Scales and Domain Knowledge. When looking at coping scales no differentiation between age groups can be made, because of the small sample of diabetics ($n = 8$). Nonetheless diabetics seem to perceive their diabetes to be as only lightly pervasive (DP: $M = 2.4$, $SD = 1.3$). The diabetics seem to have a high desire for information and control (DCI: $M = 4.7$, $SD = 0.7$) as well as trust in their doctor's competence (TDC: $M = 4.1$, $SD = 0.5$).

Diabetics were very well informed about diabetes and rather fairly informed about their obesity (IFG: $M = 3.9$, $SD = 0.3$, IFO: $M = 2.5$, $SD = 0.2$). This is not unusual because all diabetics were type-1 diabetics.

Correlation analysis showed that both IFO and IFG did not correlate with any other measures, except with themselves ($r = .824$, $p < .05$). The duration of diabetes only interacted also interacted with the informedness of obesity related factors ($r = -.793$, $p < .05$). The longer a participant has had diabetes (early onset) the less he was informed about obesity, which is externally valid, since obesity related information is of more interest to late-onset diabetes. Furthermore we found that diabetes pervasiveness did correlate with perceived cognitive deficits ($r = .812$, $p < .05$). All other measures did not correlate with coping style scales.

Further analyses of these variables are not performed.

Task Performance. Task performance was determined by both task success rate for effectiveness and time on task as efficiency. Effectiveness seems to be very high in the younger age group over all tasks (see Fig. 5). The older age group seems in contrast to have more problems with the later tasks. The only tasks that seems to make no difference between age groups are task one and task five. Correlation analysis shows that tasks three ($r = -.473$, $p < .05$) and four ($r = -.450$, $p < .05$) do correlate significantly with age. The older a user is the less effective he is at completing these tasks.

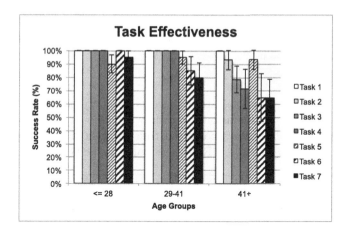

Fig. 5. Marginal means of effectiveness for all tasks in percent over age. Error bars denote standard error. Figure from [7].

When looking at efficiency for individual task (see Fig. 6) individual task length becomes visible. Task five seems to take the most time from all participants, while task two seem to take the least.

As only the last three tasks are measured as a performance experiment, reliability of these three task as a scale was assess with a Cronbach's $\alpha = .734$. This indicates that the last three tasks can be used as one scale. Because these three individual measurements ($\mathrm{ToT}_5, \mathrm{ToT}_6, \mathrm{ToT}_7$) have different maxima and minima, the geometric mean is chosen as a function to unite these variables to a total time on task (ToT) as follow:

$$ToT = \sqrt[3]{ToT_5 * ToT_6 * ToT_7}$$

The average ToT a user takes is $M = 10\,s$ ($SD = 3.71\,s$). The minimal ToT is 4.4 s and the maximal ToT is 20.8 s.

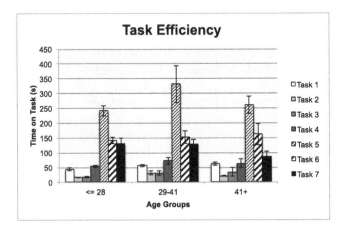

Fig. 6. Efficiency measure marginal means for all tasks over age. Error bars denote standard error. Figure from [7].

It seems necessary to incorporate the success rate into the efficiency measurement, because users could be faster at a task, when they simply skipped certain elements of a task. Therefore a corrected time on task (CTOT) is calculated using the effectiveness measure (SR=success rate) of the last three tasks.

$$CToT = \sqrt[3]{ToT_5/SR_5 * ToT_6/SR_6 * ToT_7/SR_7}$$

This measure shows a mean of 14.4 s ($SD = 14$) with a minimum of 4.4 s and a maximum of 62.4 s.

Univariate ANOVA analysis indicates that age groups do not differ in regard to efficiency ($F(2, 25) = 2.245$, n.s.). Correlation analysis confirms this ($r = .306$, $p = .14$).

9.2   Effects on Performance

When trying to understand how performance is determined multiple linear regression analyses are performed.

First a model for success rate is generated using age, diabetes duration, technical expertise and computer self-efficacy as possible predictors. Interestingly only a model with a single predictor remained significant. The model used expertise in household technology as a predictor and was able to explain 27% (adj. $r^2 = .27$) more variance than the scale mean ($F(1, 17) = 7.714$, $p < .05$). The constant term showed a coefficient of $B = 2.185$ ($SEB = 0.473$) and the predictor EHT showed a coefficient of $B = -0.265$ ($SEB = 0.09$) and a standardized slope of $\beta = -.559$. This means that household technology actually influences effective negatively.

Secondly a model of corrected time on task was generated using the same predictors as in the last regression. A model using EHT and CSE as predictors was shown to explain 47% (adj. $r^2 = .47$) more variance than the scale mean ($F(2, 15) = 8.52$, $p < .01$). Expertise with household technology again showed negative influence on performance while computer self-efficacy showed positive effects (see Table 1). Variance inflation was negligible ($VIF = 1.036$). The only downside of this model is the relatively high standard error of the constant term. Removing the weakest predictor from the model, did

Table 1. Linear regression table for corrected time on task. All predictors increased the explained variance significantly. Used from [7].

Predictor	Unstandardized coefficients		Standardized slope
	B	SEB	β
(Constant)	−32.476	37.140	
EHT	16.952	5.732	.531
CSE	−8.508	3.711	−.412

The only downside of this model is the relatively high standard error of the constant term. Removing the weakest predictor (i.e. CSE) from the model, did not decrease the standard error to a drastically more acceptable size ($SEB = 32.7$), while at the same time the explained variance decreases to 33% (adj. $r^2 = .33$, $F(1, 16) = 9.358$, $p < .01$).

9.3   Pen Evaluation

After the experiment was finished it was of high interest to find out, how much participants liked the digital pen-based diabetes diary. We based the assessment on a TAM model using both perceived ease of use and perceived usefulness as predictors for the behavioral intention. Furthermore we wanted to investigate how technical expertise influenced behavioral intention.

We measured perceived ease of use and usefulness for nine features and combined them into two scales. Reliability was analyzed using Cronbach's α. Perceived ease of use showed excellent reliability with a Cronbach's $\alpha = .914$, similarly to perceived usefulness, which showed also an excellent reliability of $\alpha = .909$. The scales are calculated as the mean of the items. The three behavioral intention items showed an acceptable reliability of $\alpha = .782$. The scale BI was calculated as the mean of these items.

When looking at how the age group influences the three scales PEU, PU, and BI (see Fig. 7), differences are hard to make out. Only perceived ease of use seems to show a difference between young and medium aged users. Though Univariate ANOVA rejects this hypothesis ($F(2, 19) = 2.373$, n.s.). In general perceived ease of use is high ($M = 5.01$, $SD = 0.75$), perceived usefulness is very high ($M = 5.44$, $SD = 0.58$) and behavioral intention is also very high ($M = 5.38$, $SD = 0.58$).

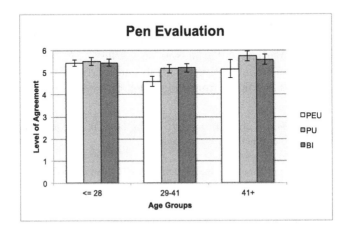

Fig. 7. Marginal means of PEU, PU, and BI over age groups. Error bars denote standard error. Figure from [7].

In order to determine what factors predict the behavioral intention a TAM based model using both PEU and PU as predictors was used. Additionally diversity factors like age, gender (dummy coded), diabetes duration, technology-expertise, and computer self-efficacy were used as predictors. Only the pure TAM based model using a two predictor model with PEU and PU as predictors was able to significantly explain more variance than the scale mean. This model was able to explain 86% (adj. $r^2 = .859$) more variance than the scale mean ($F(2, 15) = 52.747$, $p < .01$). This is a very large effect. The perceived usefulness was about three times stronger in predicting the behavioral intention than the perceived ease of use (see Table 2). Both predictors had a positive influence on the behavioral intention.

9.4   Qualitative Insights

During the experiments positive feedback about the pen in general was extensive. Participants were surprised that a pen was able to "understand" what they were writing. One participant (female, 55 years) was very reluctant to take part in the experiment because, she "hate[s] all technology." She said:

Table 2. Linear regression results for behavioral intention. Used from [7].

Predictor	Unstandardized coefficients		Standardized slope
	B	SEB	β
(Constant)	−0.04	0.54	
PEU	0.210	0.123	.244
PU	0.798	0.155	.734

"Stay away from me with this nonsense. All you engineers should try to learn that normal people like me cannot use these complicated devices."[3]

After persuading her to take part in the experiment and using the pen she stated that she loved the friendly interaction with the pen, and the pen actually felt good in her hand. She would like to have pens be as heavy as this one, as normal pens were to tiny for her to use.

Most participants showed similar reactions. Even the non-diabetic participants were delighted with the pen usage and in particular with the feeling that technology could "understand" them. Some even asked whether they could buy a pen for non-diabetic related tasks.

10   Discussion

The results (see Fig. 8) from our user study are exciting because some of the results we received were very much unexpected, while others are very expected. We could show that age has a negative impact on self-efficacy and expertise in household technologies (support of H_1 and H_2), while it has no impact on computerized technology (as opposed to H_2). This could have been a sample effect. Our sample was rather small and the participants that we had were very technically adept.

Even more exciting, however, is that the expertise with household technologies has a negative effect on the belief in self-efficacy with the pen (disagreeing with H_3), whereas computer self-efficacy has a positive effect (supporting H_3). This means people who feel less confident in using technology felt that using our digital diary was relatively easy. A possible explanation could be that the pen is operated manually and no computer-typical forms of interaction, e.g. buttons, are necessary to create a diary entry. Strangely, efficiency and effectiveness have no impact on the evaluation of use (PEU and PU). Normally, users rate technology better when their usage of it is effective.

An influence of the experience with diabetes, by duration of the disease on the one hand, and by domain knowledge on the other hand, could not be found with regard to effectiveness (rejecting H_4). This could mean that the diary was as easy to use for diabetics as it was for non-diabetics. This could have been caused by the fact that the help function was implemented in great detail and explained many features during use in the experiment.

---

[3] Translated from german.

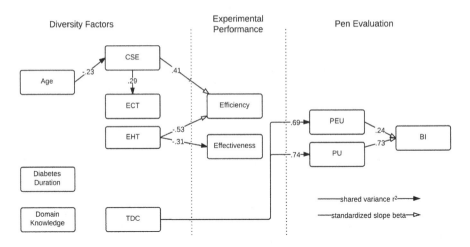

Fig. 8. Visual representation of results, showing both correlation and linear regression data. The minus sign in front of a value indicates the direction of the correlation, and is not result of an complex number squared. It was added after squaring. Figure from [7].

No effect of efficiency or effectiveness in the use of the pen was found on its evaluation (rejecting H_5). This effect was expected and similar findings can be found in the experiment by Calero Valdez et al. [33].

The influence of perceived ease of use and perceived usefulness on the intention to use was as strong as predicted by theory (supporting H_6). Both increase the intention to use. As the ease of use was generally the strength of the association with the behavioral intention was lower than the association of perceived usefulness. The usefulness showed a similar distribution as the ease of use. Ultimately, usefulness remained the more important criterion. Ease of use can thus be described as a necessary condition, while usefulness poses as a sufficient condition for acceptance.

Our findings strengthen the idea, that personalized medicine—here in the form of adaptive digital therapy—is not out of reach even for elderly users. When input technology and the output of artificial intelligence is transmitted through familiar channels (here a pen and voice), technology becomes less of a burden and more of an assistant [45].

One of the future research questions would be to investigate how data that is recorded in such diabetes assistants should be shared with doctors. How should it be utilized for recommending different healthcare options and therapies? Such questions must bee seen in the light of questions about data privacy [46] and data utilization, to truly include the user in their answers. Whether future digital diabetes assistants are hidden in pens, in voice assistants such as Alexa or even present as physical robots [47], the questions of acceptance have to be asked and re-asked to address the changing perspective on technology and artificial intelligence.

A truly personal assistant only communicates as the patient needs it. Acceptance will always require addressing the questions: when, what, how, and where from a users perspective [48]?

10.1   Limitations and Future Work

In this work we triangulated how to optimally design a digital diabetes diary using both qualitative and quantitative methods. This helped to understand the requirements of users, particular older users. Still, evaluation of these recommendations in long term studies is necessary. Using this small sample and this short usage term, extrapolation of usage intention is not feasible.

Future work should also investigate how different learning trajectories affect performance. Users in our study showed an improved during the first tasks, and long term studies will have to factor this in.

Future research should also elaborate on the influence of different personality types. We found an influence of trust in doctors competence in the rating of ease of use. This could have been caused by the setting in the doctors clinic. Other personality factors could also influence how users evaluate such a device.

Understanding how different users with different technical abilities handle such sensitive technology such as digital diabetes diaries is informative when designing products for the aging and frail cohorts of society. Further, by understanding what features are regarded as useful and easy to use by what sub-population of the users, developing customized solutions for different patients groups becomes possible. In a sense, Industrie 4.0 and mass customization could even allow that the users themselves start designing such devices. However, this still requires the development of methods that allow non-technologically savvy users to formulate their requirements and needs. When such methods exist, mass customization of health technology—in a sense personalized medicine— may finally become available.

Acknowledgements. We would like to thank Hennadiy Verkh for the development of the software prototype. Furthermore we would like to thank the participants for taking part in the study and sharing their insights. We would also like to thank the anonymous reviewers for their input on a previous version of this article.

References

1. Atzori, L., Iera, A., Morabito, G.: The internet of things: a survey. Comput. Netw. **54**, 2787–2805 (2010)
2. Davis, G.B.: Anytime/anyplace computing and the future of knowledge work. Commun. ACM **45**, 67–73 (2002)
3. Holzinger, A., Dorner, S., Födinger, M., Valdez, A.C., Ziefle, M.: Chances of increasing youth health awareness through mobile wellness applications. In: Leitner, G., Hitz, M., Holzinger, A. (eds.) USAB 2010. LNCS, vol. 6389, pp. 71–81. Springer, Heidelberg (2010). https://doi.org/10.1007/978-3-642-16607-5_5

4. Scheermesser, M., Kosow, H., Rashid, A., Holtmann, C.: User acceptance of pervasive computing in healthcare: main findings of two case studies. In: Second International Conference on Pervasive Computing Technologies for Healthcare, PervasiveHealth 2008, pp. 205–213. IEEE (2008)

5. Klack, L., Schmitz-Rode, T., Wilkowska, W., Kasugai, K., Heidrich, F., Ziefle, M.: Integrated home monitoring and compliance optimization for patients with mechanical circulatory support devices. Ann. Biomed. Eng. **39**, 2911 (2011)

6. Holzinger, A., et al.: Mobile computing is not always advantageous: lessons learned from a real-world case study in a hospital. In: Teufel, S., Min, T.A., You, I., Weippl, E. (eds.) CD-ARES 2014. LNCS, vol. 8708, pp. 110–123. Springer, Cham (2014). https://doi.org/10.1007/978-3-319-10975-6_8

7. Calero Valdez, A., Ziefle, M.: Acceptance of a digital paper-based diabetes diary. In: 4th International Conference on Information and Communication Technologies for Ageing Well and e-Health (2018)

8. Bloom, D.E., Canning, D.: Global demographic change: dimensions and economic significance. Working Paper 10817, National Bureau of Economic Research (2004)

9. Bundesamt, Statistisches: Datenreport Deutschland 2011 (2011)

10. Siebert, H.: Economic Policy for Aging Societies - Global Prevalence of Diabetes. Springer, Heidelberg (2002). https://www.springer.com/us/book/9783540432272

11. Hader, C., et al.: Diagnostik, therapie und Verlaufskontrolle des diabetes mellitus im alter. Diabetes Stoffwechsel **13**, S31–S56 (2004)

12. Rosenbloom, A.L., Joe, J.R., Young, R.S., Winter, W.E.: Emerging epidemic of type 2 diabetes in youth. Diabetes Care **22**, 345–354 (1999)

13. Hien, P., Böhm, B.: Diabetes-Handbuch: eine Anleitung für Praxis und Klinik. Springer, Heidelberg (2007). https://doi.org/10.1007/978-3-540-68174-8

14. Chen, Y.: Take it personally: accounting for individual difference in designing diabetes management systems. In: Proceedings of the 8th ACM Conference on Designing Interactive Systems, pp. 252–261. ACM (2010)

15. Stone, A.A., Shiffman, S., Schwartz, J.E., Broderick, J.E., Hufford, M.R.: Patient non-compliance with paper diaries. BMJ **324**, 1193–1194 (2002)

16. Yeung, S.E., Fischer, A.L., Dixon, R.A.: Exploring effects of type 2 diabetes on cognitive functioning in older adults. Neuropsychology **23**, 1 (2009)

17. Brands, A.M., et al.: A detailed profile of cognitive dysfunction and its relation to psychological distress in patients with type 2 diabetes mellitus. J. Int. Neuropsychol. Soc. **13**, 288–297 (2007)

18. Gorman, C.A., et al.: DEMS—a second generation diabetes electronic management system. Comput. Methods Programs Biomed. **62**, 127–140 (2000)

19. Lutes, K.D., Baggili, I.M.: Diabetic e-management system (DEMS). In: Third International Conference on Information Technology: New Generations 2006, ITNG 2006, pp. 619–624. IEEE (2006)

20. Kerkenbush, N.L.: A comparison of self-documentation in diabetics: electronic versus paper diaries. In: AMIA Annual Symposium Proceedings, vol. 2003, p. 887. American Medical Informatics Association (2003)

21. Broderick, J.E., Stone, A.A.: Paper and electronic diaries: too early for conclusions on compliance rates and their effects-comment on green, rafaeli, bolger, shrout, and reis (2006). Psychol. Methods **11**, 106–111 (2006)

22. Forjuoh, S.N., Reis, M.D., Couchman, G.R., Ory, M.G.: Improving diabetes self-care with a PDA in ambulatory care. Telemed. e-Health **14**, 273–279 (2008)

23. Duke, D.L., Thorpe, C., Mahmoud, M., Zirie, M.: Intelligent diabetes assistant: using machine learning to help manage diabetes. In: IEEE/ACS International Con-

ference on Computer Systems and Applications, AICCSA 2008, pp. 913–914. IEEE (2008)

24. Tani, S., Marukami, T., Matsuda, A., Shindo, A., Takemoto, K., Inada, H.: Development of a health management support system for patients with diabetes mellitus at home. J. Med. Syst. **34**, 223–228 (2010)

25. Kollipara, S., Silverstein, J.H., Marschilok, K.: Diabetes technologies and their role in diabetes management. Am. J. Health Educ. **40**, 292–297 (2009)

26. Burke, L.E., et al.: Self-monitoring dietary intake: current and future practices. J. Ren. Nutr. **15**, 281–290 (2005)

27. Burke, L.E., et al.: The effect of electronic self-monitoring on weight loss and dietary intake: a randomized behavioral weight loss trial. Obesity **19**, 338–344 (2011)

28. Arning, K., Ziefle, M.: Understanding age differences in PDA acceptance and performance. Comput. Hum. Behav. **23**, 2904–2927 (2007)

29. Ziefle, M.: The influence of user expertise and phone complexity on performance, ease of use and learnability of different mobile phones. Behav. Inf. Technol. **21**, 303–311 (2002)

30. Alagöz, F., Calero Valdez, A., Wilkowska, W., Ziefle, M., Dorner, S., Holzinger, A.: From cloud computing to mobile internet, from user focus to culture and hedonism: the crucible of mobile health care and wellness applications. In: 2010 5th International Conference on Pervasive Computing and Applications (ICPCA), pp. 38–45. IEEE (2010)

31. Alagöz, F., Ziefle, M., Wilkowska, W., Valdez, A.C.: Openness to accept medical technology - a cultural view. In: Holzinger, A., Simonic, K.-M. (eds.) USAB 2011. LNCS, vol. 7058, pp. 151–170. Springer, Heidelberg (2011). https://doi.org/10.1007/978-3-642-25364-5_14

32. Gregory, C.L.: "But i want a real book": an investigation of undergraduates' usage and attitudes toward electronic books. Ref. User Serv. Q., 266–273 (2008)

33. Calero Valdez, A., Ziefle, M., Horstmann, A., Herding, D., Schroeder, U.: Effects of aging and domain knowledge on usability in small screen devices for diabetes patients. In: Holzinger, A., Miesenberger, K. (eds.) USAB 2009. LNCS, vol. 5889, pp. 366–386. Springer, Heidelberg (2009). https://doi.org/10.1007/978-3-642-10308-7_26

34. Calero Valdez, A., Ziefle, M., Horstmann, A., Herding, D., Schroeder, U.: Task performance in mobile and ambient interfaces. does size matter for usability of electronic diabetes assistants? In: 2010 International Conference on Information Society (i-Society), pp. 514–521. IEEE (2010)

35. Calero Valdez, A., Ziefle, M., Horstmann, A., Herding, D., Schroder, U.: Mobile devices used for medical applications: insights won from a usability study with diabetes patients. Int. J. Digit. Soc. (IJDS) **2**, 337–346 (2011)

36. Gwizdka, J., Louie, J., Fox, M.S.: EEN: a pen-based electronic notebook for unintrusive acquisition of engineering design knowledge. In: Proceedings of the 5th Workshop on Enabling Technologies: Infrastructure for Collaborative Enterprises, pp. 40–46. IEEE (1996)

37. Pettersson, M.P.: Reconstruction of virtual raster (2005). US Patent 6,929,183

38. Kauranen, P.: The ANOTO pen - why light scattering matters (2004)

39. Carlson, J.K.: What do you do with a digital pen? In: Assistive Technologies: Concepts, Methodologies, Tools, and Applications, pp. 544–548. IGI Global (2014)

40. Davis, F.D.: Perceived usefulness, perceived ease of use, and user acceptance of information technology. MIS Q. **13**, 319–340 (1989)

41. Venkatesh, V., Morris, M.G., Davis, G.B., Davis, F.D.: User acceptance of information technology: toward a unified view. MIS Q. **27**, 425–478 (2003)
42. Venkatesh, V., Zhang, X., Sykes, T.A.: "Doctors do too little technology": a longitudinal field study of an electronic healthcare system implementation. Inf. Syst. Res. **22**, 523–546 (2011)
43. Venkatesh, V., Bala, H.: Technology acceptance model 3 and a research agenda on interventions. Decis. Sci. **39**, 273–315 (2008)
44. Beier, G.: Kontrollüberzeugungen im Umgang mit Technik: ein Persönlichkeitsmerkmal mit Relevanz für die Gestaltung technischer Systeme (2003). http://dissertation.de
45. Calero Valdez, A., Ziefle, M., Verbert, K., Felfernig, A., Holzinger, A.: Recommender systems for health informatics: state-of-the-art and future perspectives. In: Holzinger, A. (ed.) Machine Learning for Health Informatics. LNCS (LNAI), vol. 9605, pp. 391–414. Springer, Cham (2016). https://doi.org/10.1007/978-3-319-50478-0_20
46. Calero Valdez, A., Ziefle, M.: The users' perspective on the privacy-utility trade-offs in health recommender systems. Int. J. Hum.-Comput. Stud. **121**, 108–121 (2018)
47. Ziefle, M., Calero Valdez, A.: Domestic robots for homecare: a technology acceptance perspective. In: Zhou, J., Salvendy, G. (eds.) ITAP 2017. LNCS, vol. 10297, pp. 57–74. Springer, Cham (2017). https://doi.org/10.1007/978-3-319-58530-7_5
48. Calero Valdez, A.: Technology Acceptance and Diabetes: User Centered Design of Small Screen Devices for Diabetes Patients. Apprimus-Verlag (2014)

Individual Factors that Influence the Acceptance of Mobile Health Apps: The Role of Age, Gender, and Personality Traits

Andreia Nunes[✉], Teresa Limpo, and São Luís Castro

Center for Psychology at University of Porto,
Faculty of Psychology and Education Sciences, University of Porto,
Porto, Portugal
andreianunes@fpce.up.pt

Abstract. Mobile health applications (mHealth apps) are aimed to help people in the management of their lifestyle or a particular disease. The main goal of these apps is to improve health outcomes, through consumers' active self-management and involvement in healthcare. In the last years, this type of technology has been attracting the interest of researchers and consumers. mHealth apps can have an important impact in peoples' lives as they may create early habits for monitoring their health through technology, which may be essential to use mHealth over time. The use of this self-management health technology is particularly relevant for elders, as these apps offer them the possibility to manage their health with autonomy. However, some resistance can characterize the acceptance of use of technology by elders. For that reason, it seems important to understand how user's behaviors are influenced by personal characteristics, preferably before they reach the elderly stage of life. The present study explored the main effects of age, gender, and personality traits on the behavioral intention to use mHealth apps, and the moderating role of age and gender in the relationship between personality traits and the behavioral intention to use mHealth apps on non-users of this type of ICT ($N = 273$, 18–65 years). Results showed that gender plays a moderating role in the relationship between two personality traits and the behavioral intention to use mHealth apps, namely extraversion and emotional stability. These findings seem relevant to develop and adjust technologies to key characteristics of target groups, and therefore to help people to improve their quality of life.

Keywords: Mobile health applications · Age · Gender · Personality · Technology acceptance

1 Introduction

In the last decades, consumers' behaviors and their lifestyle have been largely influenced by the fast progress and mass dissemination of mobile devices [1]. Nowadays, there are an abundant number of applications, offered for free and easily accessible. A very popular

© Springer Nature Switzerland AG 2019
P. D. Bamidis et al. (Eds.): ICT4AWE 2018, CCIS 982, pp. 167–179, 2019.
https://doi.org/10.1007/978-3-030-15736-4_9

group of applications are "mobile health applications", known as mHealth, including several utilities that are useful to monitor health-related behaviors and diseases.

However, the fast-paced development and current importance of Information and Communication Technology (ICT) contrasts with the slow-paced implementation of scientific studies. Indeed, research into ICT can barely keep up with consumer demands and the digital industry [2]. Therefore, despite the numerous mHealth applications (hereafter, apps) available in the market, little is known about the factors that lead people to use them. This is particularly evident in the development of apps within the health domain, that represents a growing steadily market over the last 10 years, with 325,000 mHealth apps available in 2017[1] [3]. Understanding the determinants of ICT acceptance is important. Indeed, if no one uses ICT, its value will be reduced.

Key factors that may influence ICT acceptance are users' characteristics, such as age, gender, and personality traits [4]. These factors may or may not facilitate the adoption of ICT. Understanding their impact on ICT acceptance may be essential to know the nature of the relationship between consumers' personal characteristics and their behavioral intention to use ICT. Consequently, it will be useful for designers and marketers to develop apps tailored to the characteristics of targeted groups [2].

Elders are a particular group that could benefit from the use of mHealth apps. New models of positive ageing based on health promotion and high-quality lifestyles have been created due to the increase in life expectancy and the consequent growth of elderly [5]. By allowing elders to monitor their health with autonomy, mHealth seems to be a very promising tool to promote their independent living and to facilitate their communication with doctors [6]. However, some difficulties in engaging with ICT may make elders reluctant to use this type of technologies [7]. Thus, it seems critical to have information on key factors that influence ICT acceptance before the elderly stage of life. By promoting the use of health apps in older and younger adults, who sooner or later will be in the elderly side of society, a long-term impact on their future lives could be achieved, creating early habits to use ICT and promoting their sustained use over time. As noted by Charness [8] the prevention of age-associated impairments and the facilitation of a healthy entrance into old age could be potentiated by the early use of ICT.

Overall, it seems that one way to promote the use of mHealth apps by elders is by prompting their use from early on, and by tailoring them to relatively stable personal characteristics. Grounded on these ideas, we conducted the present study aimed to examine the moderating role of age and gender in the relationship between personality traits and the behavioral intention to use mHealth apps on non-users of this type of ICT (18-65 years). This paper represents an extension of a previous work presented in the Conference ICT4AWE [9]. Here, we refined the criteria for including participants and used more sophisticated statistical procedures.

---

[1] Research2Guidance is a market research company focused in the mobile app eco-system. For more information: https://research2guidance.com/product/mhealth-economics-2017-current-status-and-future-trends-in-mobile-health/.

2 State of the Art

2.1 Technology Acceptance

The knowledge from multiple disciplines is required to understand the relationship between consumers' characteristics and ICT use. Among these, psychology is a critical one. The focus on the psychological functioning of consumers, psychology may help to create useful technologies tailored to users' individual needs and characteristics [5].

Several models explaining factors that influence individuals' acceptance and use of ICT have been developed over the last two decades [4, 10, 11]. Based on the premise that there is a strong relationship between behavioral intentions and actual behaviors, these models were inspired by psychological and sociological theories (e.g., Theory of Reasoned Action) [12] aimed to explain why people behave in a certain way [4]. The Technology Acceptance Model (TAM) [13–15] and the Unified Theory of Acceptance and Use of Technology (UTAUT) [10] appear as the two most relevant and studied ICT acceptance models, and have been applied in several fields such as education and organizational settings [1]. In general, these models assume that behavioral intention to use, and effective use of ICT, are influenced by a set of ICT acceptance determinants, namely performance expectancy, effort expectancy, social influence, and facilitating conditions [16]. Performance expectancy refers to individuals' perception of the benefits related to ICT use; effort expectancy denotes the extent to which individuals see a particular ICT as easy to use; social influence refers to the extent to which consumers perceive that important others, such as family and friends, believe they should use ICT; and facilitating conditions focuses on consumers' perception of the technical support available to perform a behavior required by the ICT [4, 11]. The effects of ICT acceptance determinants on behavioral intention to use ICT can be either amplified or constrained by several moderators, such as age, gender, experience, and voluntariness [11, 17].

As TAM and UTAUT models were more oriented to organizational settings and the non-voluntary use of ICT by workers (e.g., as part of a job task), recently researchers start focusing on the acceptance of ICT used by consumers on a voluntary basis [4]. Thus, the UTAUT model was developed to cover the voluntary consumers 'behavior. Motivation, price value, and habits were determinants added to this new model, and age and gender were highlighted as relevant moderators for the association between ICT acceptance determinants and behavioral intention to use ICT [4]. Still, to understand the willingness to use ICT, it is also important to consider other user's characteristics, such as those captured by personality traits [18]. Little effort has been made to incorporate personality traits into a comprehensive approach to ICT acceptance, despite the recent interest from ICT developers to consider users' characteristics in ICT' development [19].

2.2 Personality and Technology

The Big-Five personality model is one of the most widely accepted models in personality research. In this model, personality characteristics are organized into five trait dimension: Extraversion, Agreeableness, Conscientiousness, Emotional Stability, and

Openness [20]. Together, these trait dimension capture the essence of personality with each dimension representing single and unique human characteristics [21]. Extraversion refers to sociability, need for stimulation, and capacity for joy. Agreeableness refers to the quality of interpersonal orientation along a continuum from compassion to antagonism. Conscientiousness refers to the individual's degree of organization, persistence, and motivation in task-and goal-directed behaviors. Emotional Stability refers to the individual's disposition in being emotionally adjusted or not. Openness refers to the need for variety, novelty, and change.

Few studies have examined the effects of the five personality traits on people's intention to use technologies [18, 19, 22, 23]. People with higher extraversion seem to have a higher degree of interaction with computers [23]. Those with high scores on agreeableness tend to cooperate more with others in adopting and use a new ICT [24]. Individuals scoring higher on conscientiousness are more careful when they evaluate the opportunities offered by technology. Moreover, scoring lower on emotionally stability was related to more reluctance in new ICT adoption [24], whereas more openness to experience were related with higher acceptance of new ICT [25].

2.3   Age, Gender, and Technology

The direct impact of age and gender on ICT use has received little attention in prior models of ICT acceptance [19]. Instead, age and gender have been studied only as moderators of the relationship between major determinants of ICT acceptance and the behavioral intention to use technologies [11].

Age was found to be a key moderator in the UTAUT model [11]. For example, performance expectancy was a stronger determinant of ICT acceptance in younger people, whereas in older people effort expectancy and facilitating conditions were more important to their ICT acceptance.

Concerning gender, performance expectancy was a stronger determinant for men's behavioral intention to use ICT, whereas for women their intentions were more influenced by effort expectancy, facilitating conditions, social influence, and previous experience with technologies [4, 11]. Thus, it seems important to take into account age and gender when examining the role of individual differences in ICT acceptance.

As age and gender seem to display a moderating role in ICT acceptance models, they seem potential moderators on the relationship between personality and behavioral intention to use ICT. In the study of the big-five dimensions have already been reported age and gender differences. For example, older adults were found to be more self-disciplined and agreeable than younger adults [26], and women scored higher on agreeableness and lower on emotional stability than men [27].

2.4   Present Study

As previous reviewed, the study of factors underlying consumer's intention to use ICT has been growing. However, few studies examined the role that personal characteristics as age, gender, and personality traits displays in such intentions, specially in what refers to mHealth apps [2]. Here, we examine the moderating role of age and gender in the relationship between personality traits and the behavioral intention to use mHealth apps on non-users of this type of ICT. We asked two major research questions. Do age, gender, and personality traits influence individuals' behavioral intention to use mHealth apps? And do age and gender moderate the effects of personality traits on individuals' behavioral intention to use mHealth apps?

3 Methodology

3.1 Participants

Three-hundred eighty-five individuals took part in this study, all native speakers of European Portuguese. We set one exclusion criteria, which was currently using mHealth apps. Based on this, we removed 67 participants from the data-analytic sample. This exclusion criteria represents a novelty to previous work [9]. In this way, we were able to analyze the acceptance of mHealth in a more homogeneous sample, only with non-users of this type of ICT, and therefore to make stronger claims about intentions to use. Additionally, 45 participants were excluded because they did not respond to at least one item of the questionnaires, resulting in a total of 273 participants. They were aged between 18 and 65 years ($M = 34.94$, $SD = 15.74$) and 76% were women. Among all participants, 6% had completed primary education (4 years), 4% upper primary education (6 years), 6% middle education (9 years), 11% secondary education (12 years); 44% were attending university, and 29% held a university degree.

3.2 Procedure and Measures

A booklet including a set of questionnaires was initially administered to undergraduates in classroom groups. After completing the questionnaires, undergraduates were asked to take an additional booklet with them and have it filled by an acquaintance or family member aged between 40 and 65 years within 15 days. This booklet included several questionnaires that were part a larger study on personality and health literacy. Only the measures relevant to the present study are described here.

To assess the Big-Five dimensions of personality we used the Ten-Item Personality Inventory (TIPI) [original version: 28; Portuguese version: 29]. TIPI includes two items —a single word or phrase—per dimension (10 items in total), and participants are asked to rate the extent to which each trait applies to themselves using a 7-point scale (1 = *strongly disagree*; 7 = *strongly agree*).

To measure the behavioral intention to use mHealth apps we used the Behavioral Intention sub-scale of the Questionnaire of Acceptance of Technology – mHealth Apps, adapted from [30]. Participants indicate their level of agreement with sentences on the potential use of mHealth apps (e.g., *Assuming I had access to health apps, I would intend to use it.*), using a 7-point scale (1 = *strongly disagree*; 7 = *strongly agree*).

4 Results

4.1 Descriptive Statistics and Correlations

Table 1 presents means and standard deviations for all predictors and outcome variables, along with the bivariate correlations between each other. Women tended to exhibit higher levels of agreeableness than men ($r = -.15$), and men tended to exhibit higher levels of emotional stability than women ($r = .24$). Older participants tended to exhibit higher levels of conscientiousness ($r = .16$), more emotional stability ($r = .23$), and more behavioral intention to use mHealth apps ($r = .19$).

Table 1. Means, standard deviations and correlations for all variables (N = 273)

Measures	Correlations							
	Age	Gender	E	A	C	ES	O	BI
1. Age								
2. Gender[a]	.27**							
3. Extraversion	.04	−.03						
4. Agreeableness	.10	−.15*	−.02					
5. Conscientiousness	.16**	−.09	.13*	.30**				
6. Emotional Stability	.23**	.24**	.21**	.21**	.17**			
7. Openness	−.09	.01	.39**	.16**	.08	.21**		
8. Behavioral Intention	.19**	−.03	.08	.09	.12*	−.002	.08	
M	34.94	0.24	4.54	6.11	5.75	3.88	5.27	4.09
SD	15.74	0.43	1.60	0.82	1.14	1.31	1.23	1.18

[a]Dummy coded, 0 = female, 1 = male. E = Extraversion, A = Agreeableness, C = Conscientiousness, ES = Emotional Stability, O = Openness, BI = Behavioral Intention. *p < .05, **p < .01, ***p < .001.

4.2 Prediction of Behavioral Intention to Use mHealth Apps

We conducted a stepwise multiple linear regression to examine the moderating role of age and gender in the relationship between personality traits and the behavioral intention to use mHealth apps. In Step 1, we entered the main effects of age, gender, and of the five personality traits (viz., extraversion, agreeableness, conscientiousness, emotional stability and openness). Contrary to a previous version presented at the Conference ICT4AWE, where age was analyzed as a continuous variable, by splitting the sample into two categories [9], age was now introduced in the regression model as a continuous variable. In Step 2, we added the two-way interactions of age and gender with each personality dimension. In Step 3, we added the three-way interactions between age, gender, and each personality trait. All variables were previously mean centered and the Process macro for SPSS was used to decompose significant interactions [31].

In Step 1, age, gender, and the five personality traits explained 7% of the variance in behavioral intention to use mHealth apps, $R^2 = .07$, $F(7, 265) = 2.65$, $p = .01$. Results showed significant main effects of age ($B = 0.01$, $p = .001$) on individuals' behavioral intention to use mHealth apps.

In Step 2, there was a significant increase of 7% in the prediction of behavioral intention to use mHealth apps with the inclusion of the two-way interactions, $\Delta R^2 = .07$, $F_{change}(11, 254) = 1.96$, $p = .03$. Results revealed significant two-way interactions between gender and two personality traits, namely, extraversion ($B = 0.30$, $p = .01$), and emotional stability ($B = -0.36$, $p = .01$).

In Step 3, the inclusion of the three-way interactions between age, gender, and each personality traits did not result in any significant increase in the amount of variance explained, $\Delta R^2 = .02$, $F_{change}(5, 249) = 1.12$, $p = .35$. For that reason, we focused on the model from Step 2, and its two-way interactions (Table 2).

Table 2. Model with all main effects and interactions of age, gender, and personality on participants' behavioral intention to use mHealth apps.

	B	SE	β	t
Constant	2.76	.72		3.84
Age	0.01	.01	.15	1.96
Gender	−0.08	.21	−.03	−0.39
Extraversion	−0.02	.06	−.03	−0.36
Agreeableness	0.06	.11	.04	0.51
Conscientiousness	0.05	.08	.05	0.65
Emotional stability	0.03	.07	.03	0.44
Openness	0.07	.08	.07	0.87
Age × Gender	0.02	.01	.17	1.96
Age × Extraversion	0.00	.003	.01	0.13
Age × Agreeableness	0.01	.01	.07	1.02
Age × Conscientiousness	−0.001	.004	−.02	−0.3
Age × Emotional stability	−0.01	.004	−.11	−1.48
Age × Openness	0.01	.004	.13	1.74
Gender × Extraversion	0.30	.12	.19	2.50*
Gender × Agreeableness	0.17	.21	.06	0.83
Gender × Conscientiousness	0.04	.15	.02	0.27
Gender × Emotional stability	−0.36	.14	−.21	−2.63**
Gender × Openness	−0.24	.16	−.12	−1.48

*p < .05, **p < .01, ***p < .001.

Below we present the results of decomposing the significant two-way interactions.

4.2.1   Gender × Extraversion

For women, extraversion did not significantly contribute to behavioral intention to use mHealth apps, $B = -0.08$, $t = 1.07$, $p = .29$. For men, we found a significant effect of extraversion on behavioral intention to use mHealth apps. Specifically, a stronger behavioral intention to use mHealth apps was found for men displaying higher levels of extraversion, $B = 0.18$, $t = 2.55$, $p = .01$ (see Fig. 1 for a graphical display).

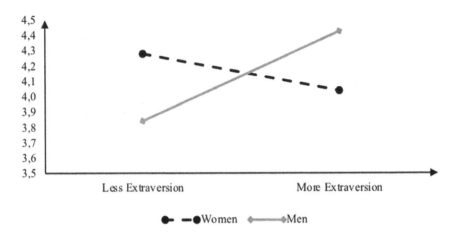

Fig. 1. Effect of extraversion on behavioral intention to use mHealth, moderated by gender.

4.2.2   Gender × Emotional Stability

For women, emotional stability did not significantly contribute to behavioral intention to use mHealth apps, $B = 0.09$, $t = 1.04$, $p = .30$. For men, we found a significant effect of emotional stability on behavioral intention to use mHealth apps. Specifically, a stronger behavioral intention to use mHealth apps was found for men displaying lower levels of emotional stability, $B = -0.22$, $t = 2.63$, $p = .01$ (see Fig. 2 for a graphical display).

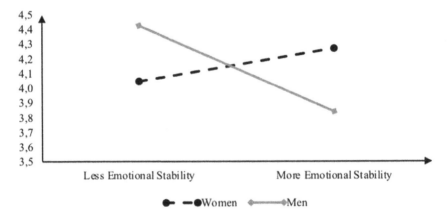

Fig. 2. Effect of emotional stability on behavioral intention to use mHealth, moderated by gender.

5   Discussion

Our main research goal was to examine the moderating role of age and gender in the relationship between personality traits and the behavioral intention to use mHealth apps on non-users of this type of ICT.

We formulated two major research questions: Do age, gender, and personality traits influence individuals' behavioral intention to use mHealth apps? And do age and gender moderate the effects of personality traits on individuals' behavioral intention to use mHealth apps? The model with main and moderation effects (i.e., two-way interactions) explained 14% of the variance in behavioral intention to use mHealth apps. As showed by moderation analysis and discussed in what follows, the significant effects of personality traits on behavioral intention to use mHealth apps were all in the form of two-way interactions, only with the moderation of gender, and not with the moderation of age.

5.1   Main Effects of Age, Gender, and Personality Traits on Behavioral Intention to Use mHealth Apps

Concerning the first research question, we found on Step 1 a main effect of age on individual's behavioral intention to use mHealth apps. Results revealed that, when entering the main effects of age, gender, and personality traits in the model, only age contributed significantly and positively to behavioral intention to use mHealth apps. This means that as individuals get older, their behavioral intention to use mHealth apps grows. However, when adding the two-way interaction between the variables on Step 2, this main effect of age was no longer significant. Indeed, on Step 2 of the regression model including main effects and two-way interactions, there were no main effects of age, gender, and personality. These results are aligned with prior findings showing no main effects of gender and personality on individuals' behavioral intention to use mHealth apps neither in younger nor in older adults [9].

Some careful is needed when interpreting the lack of these main effects. Research into ICT acceptance has barely considered the unique effects of age, gender, and personality traits to behavioral intention. Instead, age and gender have been mainly considered as antecedents of determinants of ICT acceptance (e.g., ease of use) or only as moderators of the relationship between these and behavioral intention [25, 32]. Within the UTAUT model, age and gender are considered important moderators [11]. The influence of personality was already shown to have no direct influence on individuals' behavioral intention to use ICT. Instead, its effect seems to occur through other ICT acceptance determinants, such as perceived usefulness, ease of use and social norms [18].

5.2   Moderating Role of Age and Gender on the Relationship Between Personality Traits and Behavioral Intention to Use mHealth Apps

Concerning the second research question, we found that age did not moderate the effects of personality traits on the behavioral intention to use mHealth apps. Instead, gender moderated the relationship between two personality traits and behavioral intention to use mHealth apps, namely, extraversion and emotional stability. Both simple slopes were significant only for men, but not for women. Specifically, among men, the extraversion effect on behavioral intention was positive, whereas the emotional stability effect on behavioral intention was negative. This indicates that more extraverted men and less emotionally stable men are more likely to use mHealth apps. This result is aligned with a previous study that compared younger and older individuals in their intention to use mHealth apps [9]. Additionally, other studies in the technology field found that the effects of personality traits on technology-related outcomes are moderated by participants' gender. For example, such an interaction was reported by Saleem et al. [33] in a study focused on computer self-efficacy. However, few studies have addressed the moderating role of gender on the relationship between personality and use of mobile apps in the health domain. Further studies are needed to corroborate our findings and deepen knowledge on their implications to the acceptance of mHealth.

Overall, personal characteristics seems to be important to have in consideration when studying ICT acceptance determinants. Indeed, individuals' intention to use ICT seems related to the affinity that they have for certain types of ICT, which is influenced by personal characteristics such as those here examined, that is, age, gender, and personality [17]. As suggested by ICT studies, individual differences may affect the adoption of new ICT [34]. Implications to the design and development of mHealth apps are brought by these findings. The development of new ICT solutions should therefore be tailored to particular segments of the population. Not only age and gender must be taken into consideration when developing apps, but also the behavioral patterns typical of the target groups. Future research should continue to explore how other personal characteristics influence ICT acceptance across lifetime, as people reach the elderly stage of life.

5.3   Limitations and Future Directions

The previously discussed findings should be considered in view of five limitations, which may guide future research. First, because data were obtained at a single time point and because this study is correlational in nature, causality inferences should be avoided. Additional research is needed to replicate reported results. Second, we did not measure the real use of mHealth apps. Instead, we focused on people that did not use mHealth apps and on their behavioural intention to use it. Future research should include users of mHealth apps, and eventually compare them with non-users. Third, due to the recruitment procedure, there was a larger representation of women than men in our sample. Future studies should aim to collect larger samples, with an equivalent number of men and women. Fourth, we did not use all the variables of the UTAUT model, specifically the ICT acceptance determinants (i.e., performance expectancy, effort expectancy, social influence, and facilitating conditions). In the future, researchers should consider adding these variables to test their interaction with age, gender, and personality traits. Finally, because ageing brings changes in diverse aspects, such as physical health, perception, cognition, and psychological functioning [8], it would be important to control for these aspects, particularly in older individuals. Along with age, gender, and personality, these personal characteristics may also play a role in the way that people use or intend to use mHealth.

6   Conclusions

Although personal factors have been receiving a growing attention from the app development industry, studies that examine the role of personal characteristics on ICT acceptance are still reduced. Our study provided additional knowledge on the role of age, gender, and personality in individuals' behavioral intention to use mHealth apps, on non-users of this type of ICT. We think that such knowledge is useful not only to develop ICT but also to adjust it to its target groups. The general resistance that elders show in accepting ICT [8] makes the promotion of mHealth in earlier stages of life particularly important to create habits to use ICT. Such habits are essential to ICT use through the lifespan and prevent possible negative health outcomes.

References

1. Huang, C., Kao, Y.: UTAUT2 based predictions of factors influencing the technology acceptance of phablets by DNP. Math. Prob. Eng. **2015**, 1–23 (2015). https://doi.org/10.1155/2015/603747
2. Boudreaux, E.D., Waring, M.E., Hayes, R.B., Sadasivam, R.S., Mullen, S., Pagoto, S.: Evaluating and selecting mobile health apps: strategies for healthcare providers and healthcare organizations. Transl. Behav. Med. **4**, 363–371 (2014). https://doi.org/10.1007/s13142-014-0293-9
3. Research2Guidance. mHealth app economics 2017/2018: how digital intruders are taking over the healthcare market (2017). https://research2guidance.com/product/mhealth-economics-2017-current-status-and-future-trends-in-mobile-health/
4. Venkatesh, V., Thong, J.Y.L., Xu, X.: Consumer acceptance and use of information technology: extending the unified theory of acceptance and use of technology. MIS Q. **36**, 157–178 (2012)
5. Demiris, G., et al.: Older adults' attitudes towards and perceptions of "smart home" technologies: a pilot study. Med. Inform. Internet Med. **29**, 87–94 (2004). https://doi.org/10.1080/14639230410001684387
6. Czaja, S.J.: Can technology empower older adults to manage their health? Generations **39**, 46–51 (2015)
7. Young, R., Willis, E., Cameron, G., Geana, M.: "Wiiing but unwilling": attitudinal barriers to adoption of home-based health information technology among older adults. Health Inform. J. **20**, 127–135 (2014). https://doi.org/10.1177/1460458213486906
8. Charness, N., Boot, W.R.: Aging and information technology use: potential and barriers. Curr. Dir. Psychol. Sci. **18**, 253–258 (2009). https://doi.org/10.1111/j.1467-8721.2009.01647.x
9. Nunes, A., Limpo, T., Castro, S.L.: Effects of age, gender, and personality on individuals' behavioral intention to use health applications. In: Bamidis, P.D., Ziefle, M., Maciaszek, L. (eds.) Proceedings of the 4th International Conference on Information and Communication Technologies for Ageing Well and e-Health, pp. 103–110. Santa Cruz - Madeira: SCITEPRESS – Science and Technology Publications (2018)
10. Davis, F.D.: A technology acceptance model for empirically testing new end-user information systems: theory and results. Ph.D., Wayne State University (1986)
11. Venkatesh, V., Morris, M.G., Davis, G.B., Davis, F.D.: User acceptance of information technology: toward unified view. MIS Q. **27**, 425–478 (2003)

12. Fishbein, M., Ajzen, I.: Belief, Attitude, Intention, and Behavior: An Introduction to Theory and Research. Addison-Wesley, Reading (1975)

13. Davis, F.D.: Perceived usefulness, perceived ease of use, and user acceptance of information technology. MIS Q. **13**, 319–340 (1989). https://doi.org/10.2307/249008

14. Venkatesh, V., Bala, H.: Technology acceptance model 3 and a research agenda on interventions. Decis. Sci. **39** (2008). https://doi.org/10.1111/j.1540-5915.2008.00192.x

15. Venkatesh, V., Davis, F.D.: A theoretical extension of the technology acceptance model: four longitudinal studies. Manage. Sci. **46**, 425–478 (2000). https://doi.org/10.1287/mnsc.46.2.186.11926

16. Venkatesh, V.: Determinants of perceived ease of use: integrating control, intrinsic motivation, and emotion into the technology acceptance model. Inf. Syst. Res. **11**, 342–365 (2000). https://doi.org/10.1287/isre.11.4.342.11872

17. Arenas-Gaitán, J., Peral-Peral, B., Ramón-Jerónimo, M.A.: Elderly and internet banking: an application of UTAUT2. J. Internet Banking Commer. **20**, 1–23 (2015)

18. Svendsen, G.B., Johnsen, J.K., Almås-Sørensen, L., Vittersø, J.: Personality and technology acceptance: the influence of personality factors on the core constructs of the technology acceptance model. Behav. Inf. Technol. **32**, 323–334 (2013). https://doi.org/10.1080/0144929X.2011.553740

19. Barnett, T., Pearson, A.W., Pearson, R., Kellermanns, F.W.: Five-factor model personality traits as predictors of perceived and actual usage of technology. Eur. J. Inf. Syst. **24**, 374–390 (2015). https://doi.org/10.1057/ejis.2014.10

20. Costa Jr., P.T., McCrae, R.R.: Revised NEO Personality Inventory (NEO-PI-R) and NEO Five-Factor Inventory (NEO- FFI) Professional Manual. Psychological Assessment Resources, Odessa (1992)

21. John, O.P., Srivastava, S.: The big-five trait taxonomy: history, measurement, and theoretical perspectives. In: Pervin, L.A., John, O.P. (eds.) Handbook of Personality: Theory and Research, 2nd edn. Guilford Press, New York (1999)

22. Nov, O., Ye, C.: Personality and technology acceptance: personal innovativeness in IT, openness and resistance to change. In: Proceedings of the 41st Annual Hawaii International Conference on System Sciences. IEEE Computer Science (2008)

23. Pocius, K.E.: Personality factors in Human-computer interaction: a review of the literature. Comput. Hum. Behav. **7**, 103–135 (1991)

24. Devaraj, S., Easley, R.F., Crant, J.M.: Research note - how does personality matter? Relating the five-factor model to technology acceptance and use. Inf. Syst. Res. **19**, 93–105 (2008). https://doi.org/10.1287/isre.1070.0153

25. McElroy, J.C., Hendrickson, A.R., Townsend, A.M., DeMarie, S.M.: Dispositional factors in internet use: personality versus cognitive style. MIS Q. **31**, 809–820 (2007)

26. Soto, C.J., John, O.P., Gosling, S.D., Potter, J.: Age differences in personality traits from 10 to 65: big five domains and facets in a large cross-sectional sample. J. Pers. Soc. Psychol. **100**, 330–348 (2011). https://doi.org/10.1037/a0021717

27. Chapman, B.P., Duberstein, P.R., Sörensen, S., Lyness, J.M.: Gender differences in five factor model personality traits in an elderly cohort: extension of robust and surprising findings to an older generation. Pers. Individ. Differ. **43**, 1594–1603 (2008)

28. Gosling, S.D., Rentfrow, P.J., Swann Jr., W.B.: A very brief measure of the big five personality domains. J. Res. Pers. **37**, 504–528 (2003). https://doi.org/10.1016/S0092-6566(03)00046-1

29. Nunes, A., Limpo, T., Lima, C.F., Castro, S.L.: Short scales for the assessment of personality traits: development and validation of the Portuguese ten-item personality inventory (TIPI). Front. Psychol. **9** (2018). https://doi.org/10.3389/fpsyg.2018.00461

30. Cimperman, M., Makovec Brenčič, M., Trkman, P.: Analyzing older users' home telehealth services acceptance behavior—applying an extended UTAUT model. Int. J. Med. Inform. **90**, 22–31 (2016). https://doi.org/10.1016/j.ijmedinf.2016.03.002
31. Hayes, A.F.: Introduction to Mediation, Moderation, and Conditional Process Analysis: A Regression-Based Perspective. The Guilford Press, New York (2013)
32. Tarhini, A., Hone, K., Liu, X.: Measuring the moderating effect of gender and age on e-learning acceptance in England: a structural equation modeling approach for an extended technology acceptance model. J. Educ. Comput. Res. **51**, 163–184 (2014). https://doi.org/10.2190/EC.51.2.b
33. Saleem, H., Beaudry, A., Croteau, A.-M.: Antecedents of computer self-efficacy: a study of the role of personality traits and gender. Comput. Hum. Behav. **27**, 1922–1936 (2011). https://doi.org/10.1016/j.chb.2011.04.017
34. Tsourela, M., Roumeliotis, M.: The moderating role of technology readiness, gender, and sex in consumer acceptance and actual use of technology-based services. J. High Technol. Manage. Res. **26**, 124–136 (2015). https://doi.org/10.1016/j.hitech.2015.09.003

Moving Ahead: Elaboration on Cumulative Effects on Urban and Suburban Transport Ecosystems by Enhancing Last Mile Mobility of Older Adults and Persons with Disabilities

Stefan H. Ruscher[1]([✉]), Andrea Ch. Kofler[2], Vincent Neumayer[1], and Johanna Renat[1]

[1] Wiener Linien GmbH & Co KG, Erdbergstraße 202, 1031 Vienna, Austria
stefanh.ruscher@gmail.com,
{vincent.neumayer,johanna.renat}@wienerlinien.at
[2] Zurich University of Applied Sciences,
Grüental, 8820 Wädenswil, Zurich, Switzerland
andrea.kofler@zhaw.ch

Abstract. Provision of fair, affordable and accessible transport is an essential objective of Smart Cities. In previous research, we outlined five action areas to enhance Last Mile Mobility for older adults and persons with disabilities. Following up, we expand our view towards a wider Smart City context, reflecting on needs of other target audiences of urban and suburban transport systems. By analyzing the effects of an enhanced Last Mile Mobility on children, adolescents and marginalized persons, we conclude to review the transport ecosystem as a whole. Based on this holistic view, we elaborate further on previously identified action areas, focusing first on the three action areas, which describe a transport system's service quality: spread of service areas, accessibility of provided services, and availability of demand-driven services. We continue to deepen our view on the potential role of paratransit services within the urban transport ecosystem (action area 4), and finally delve into policy needs and recommendations to maximize Last Mile mobility in Smart Cities (action area 5). We conclude our work with a suggestion for future pilot implementation based on our findings.

Keywords: Intermodal mobility · Accessibility · Last Mile transport · Public transport · Paratransit

1 Introduction

The provision of fair, affordable and accessible mobility is commonly understood as one of the core tasks of Smart Cities [1]. With the European Accessibility Act [2] outlining a special focus on passenger transport, especially public transport operators are required to improve the accessibility of mobility services in urban and suburban areas. A core challenge for the stakeholders in public transport is the coverage of the so-called "Last Mile", describing the distance between a public transport station and the

© Springer Nature Switzerland AG 2019
P. D. Bamidis et al. (Eds.): ICT4AWE 2018, CCIS 982, pp. 180–195, 2019.
https://doi.org/10.1007/978-3-030-15736-4_10

ultimate destination of a trip [3], which typically involves other forms of mobility, like walking, biking or a car ride. These modes of transport require a certain level of physical or cognitive ability. Therefore, when considering the accessibility of a transport system, the importance of an accessible Last Mile transport cannot be underrated.

In order to tackle the challenge of such an accessible Last Mile transport service provision, we first investigated the chances to enhance Last Mile mobility for older adults and persons with disabilities in Vienna, Austria, and Zurich, Switzerland [1]. Our work focused primarily on current shortcomings in the available mobility service offers, on potential gains for older adults derived from the services, and on suggestions for actions to be taken in order to enhance personal mobility. Specifically, we proposed five action areas: (1) to expand service areas, (2) to establish on-demand services, (3) to improve service accessibility, (4) to integrate medical shuttles into the public transport network, and (5) to foster the establishment of a policy framework [1]. We concluded that public transport operators play the key roles in the implementation of such actions, without yet delving into the needs of all passengers and customers.

The design of accessible products and services is generally accepted to be related to the overall customer experience [4–6]. As the public transport's "product" is to provide mobility to all citizens alike, we identified the need to expand our research on the accessible Last Mile mobility towards further customer groups as well. By doing so, further effects like the customers' social inclusion or minimization of marginalization should be analyzed, reflecting upon mutual benefits as well as potential conflicts arising from the needs of different customer segments and transport service operators.

Subsequently we explore potential user groups, who, besides older adults and persons with disabilities, would also benefit from advances in the three service-quality related action areas proposed before (expanded service area, established on-demand services and improved service accessibility) [1]. Then we extend the scope to the analysis of the service quality of transport systems, extending the findings with the requirements by the stakeholders towards an inclusive transport ecosystem. We proceed by investigating the stakeholder groups' communication and information needs within the ecosystem with the aim of enabling an enhancement of the overall mobility within transport ecosystems. Going a step beyond, we evaluate, based on our findings, the potential role of medical shuttles services – also described as paratransit [7] – within the transport ecosystem. This refers to our proposed fourth action area. Finally, contributing to the fifth action area (policy framework), we make concrete suggestions for an expanded customer-centered view on the proposed transport ecosystem. Based on our analyses we conclude by making suggestions for future activities to improve transport ecosystems.

2 Potential User Groups

Our previous research was originated from a Smart City context, but focused primarily on the benefits of demand-driven mobility services to cover the Last Mile in an AAL (Active and Assisted Living) context [1] - not yet transferring the findings back into a wider context. To tackle this shortcoming, we explored additional stakeholder groups within a Smart City context, who might face limitation in their mobility, which not directly results from a jeopardized health condition or impairment.

Lubitow et al. [8] criticize that transportation infrastructure is "oriented toward an 'ideal rider' who is an economically stable, able-bodied, white, male commuter" [8]. There are, however, many others, who rely on a transportation system, which offers accessibility, affordability, and individualized mobility services. The latter can be shared mobility services.

A starting point for finding potential beneficiaries of shared mobility concepts can be their articulation in previous research in the AAL domain, where, besides decline in physical and mental abilities, also the limiting effects of marginalization on older adults is described [9]. Yet, marginalization and poverty do not only affect older adults. Younger mobility groups e.g. kids and students, mobility groups with reduced budgets or people in distinct living situations e.g. parents travelling with their children and in need for strollers, and people with sensory and/or physical impairment would also gain from a more affordable and accessible transportation system. Both, pricing and accessibility are overall societal issues, especially in urban and suburban areas, where people depend upon a sufficient public transportation system. Users would benefit from a wide spectrum of mobility services, which also helps them to reduce transport costs. Affordable and easily accessible mobility is crucial for marginalized residents in order to participate in society and to stay active and independent [10].

Furthermore, Quodomine [11] underlines that public transportation is of similar importance for younger and older adults, as both use public transportation in lack of alternatives and financial means. Additionally, public transportation mobility provides more and more services as add-ons. Younger adults appreciate services like free Wi-Fi. The study also revealed that younger adults still consider public transportation more sustainable compared to going by car not the least for ecological reasons. The negative perception of public transportation by this user group is constantly decreasing. When it comes to the older adults, public transportation is favored because of economic reasons and decreasing driving capacity [11]. As for older adults and persons with impairments, enhanced last-mile services also improve mobility for adolescents.

Finally, safety in terms of safe and secured infrastructure is an issue not to be underestimated. Lubitow et al. [8] describe women sharing their negative experiences when riding buses and their children injured while the bus drivers not taking care of them. Obviously, safe and secure transportation infrastructure is a key concern and not to be underestimated, when it comes to the different user groups with their specific needs in this domain.

Even when discussed in a broader context, Lavadinho [12] clearly confirms the need for transportation providers to become more than just enablers for people to get from A to B. As stated above, the accessibility to Wi-Fi makes a bus or train more than just another mean of transportation. She summarizes: The "added value of the transportation system derives as much from whichever activities can be deployed along the way than from reaching the final destination. A new mind-set is therefore needed, where the success of city-access policies regarding public transport is measured by different metrics" [12]. These effects of enhanced means of transportation with regard to their customer- and ultimately stakeholder-satisfaction can also be observed with regard to enhanced station infrastructure (e.g. bus/tram stops providing Wi-Fi, snack-machines, shelter, sitting possibilities etc.) [13]. Younger generations can expect further positive side effects: Stone et al. [14] report that enhancing independent mobility for children has a preventive health effect, as improvements in personal mobility correlate with higher physical activities, as they are more likely to roam the city and participate in physical activities.

When considering these customer segments, it is obvious, that, like mobility itself, their way-finding too is more than just getting from A to B. It is about orientation, emotions, and customer satisfaction. Customers typically also evaluate their routes based on whether they feel safe and comfortable. Referring to a wide field of research, Meurer et al. [15] describe mobility as something that has spatial as well as place related dimensions. In this sense "spatial" refers to people moving around within cities, suburbs or other clearly defined environments and to terms of geographical dimensions. "Place" on the other hand refers to emotional ties, social interaction and interdependencies. A neighborhood is considered to be a place in that people have built up social networks and where they are emotionally and socially embedded. They report, that for older adults mobility in particularly has a social aspect, that it is also about interaction with others.

Similarly, Stone et al. [14] report that the social situation in neighborhoods has an influence on the mobility behavior and patterns of children. In summary, social interactions as well as the physical environment allow people to have very different mobility experiences; these experiences and expectations are affecting how they move in space. With their research, carried out in Germany in 2016 with 19 older adults, Meurer et al. [15] attempted to learn about way-finding practices and how these can be better supported by assistive technologies. The study provides insights on various different levels. Most prominently, they show that depending on the purpose of mobility, way-finding varies. They identified five different mobility situations with distinct way-finding practices: (1) weekly routines (e.g. to see their grand-children, to go to the sports club), (2) first time journeys (e.g. to see a specialist), (3) visits of beloved and attached places (e.g. a church, a park), (4) places of specific kinds (e.g. the supermarket, a restaurant) and (5) when they purposely do ridesharing. From a mobility and assisted technology perspective, it is important that they might always take the same modes of public transport for mobility situations 1 to 4. Yet, they are differently motivated and need different support and information. From a mobility and assisted technology perspective, it is important to note, that due to differently motivated mobility activities different support and information is expected. At one moment, it can be the information on the schedule, vehicle accessibility and maps, at another moment it can be a need for navigation or safety [15].

By looking at older adults and their mobility reasoning we learn that this group accesses places and uses means of transportation with distinct mind-sets and capabilities, which might vary depending on where they intend to go, how familiar they are with the place and how much support they need. Compared to other user groups, older adults create "new rhythmic mobility patterns" [15], which differ from those of commuters and students, as they visit different places at different times because of their daily routines. Therefore, addressing transportation issues for older adults also means to look at their specific transportation paths and radiuses [15]. The challenge however lays in a transportation system that deals not only with the older adults mobility behavior but also with the more flexible and ever-changing one of other users with their distinct expectations and optimizes the overall benefit to all stakeholders at any time and place.

3   Enhancement of Transport Service Quality

To address all the customer needs of older adults, younger people, persons with disabilities, and marginalized groups of people, the transport service logic needs to be more serenely analyzed. Therefore, hereinafter three action areas are discussed in more detail. Firstly, the service areas, which need to spread across urban and suburban spaces; secondly, demand-driven services, which need to be established to cover off-peak loads in a sustainable way; and thirdly, the overall accessibility of the transportation services provided. Subsequently, we will elaborate those areas in greater depth, outlining their significance to as well as implications for a transport ecosystem.

As pointed out in our first action area before, private mobility service providers usually use a pre-defined zone of operation in city centers, limited to those urban areas, which have the highest commuter and therefore customer density [1]. Yet, many older adults are living in the outer, suburban districts, where the public transport offering is limited. In Vienna for example, more than 20% of the population in the 13th, 19th and 23rd district are 64 years or older, with the majority of inhabitants being 40 years and older [16]. Leading bike and car sharing services in Vienna are primarily available around the city center, where the subway also operates [1]. In the outer districts, where only a few bus lines are available, hardly any sharing opportunity can be found. As proposed, these service areas need to be expanded towards suburban districts [1], and even further to rural areas [17] to ensure available and accessible mobility.

An expansion of operation zones for sharing services would require innovative business models to cope with the associated higher costs for relocation or the increased number of vehicles needed to retain the availability. Predicting the demand is also becoming more difficult "as fewer customers are using cars more infrequently, as it is likely for older adults and persons with disabilities in suburban areas" [1]. Nevertheless, this might result in a higher price as the service is carried out beyond the current service area. Such considerations underline the importance of an integration of private operators in the regional tariff models as a requirement to offer flexible and affordable mobility outside of the city centers.

As reported before [1], in the greater Zurich area, public transportation networks are well developed; train and bus services are well coordinated. The streetcar network is in the process to be expanded into the suburban areas. In combination with the city bus system, it provides users an extensive public transportation system. The 'Travel Time Map' provides a digital service. The user adds a departure point, the maximum journey and walking time [18]. As a user, you are offered advanced travel options, you learn about travel hubs, and you are informed about traffic routes and costs. The service is not only offered for the Zurich area, but is available for all of Switzerland, also including touristic sites. Within Switzerland the focus of actions however must be on the periurban areas, describing those areas located between urban and rural areas. Recent surveys for Switzerland confirm that 66% commute as either drivers or passengers to urban areas [19]. Based on their data Marconi and Schaad [19] further summarize that 45% of urban households within Switzerland benefit from a very good or good public transport offering, which contrasts with only 4% in the periurban areas. The authors conclude that motorized individual car transportation is still the preferred mean of transport for commuters when traveling from a periurban area to work, and that the comparatively underdeveloped public transportation network services in the periurban area results in a high number of car holders. This of course leaves us with the question of what happens if people no longer are capable to drive their own cars to see a doctor downtown, meet friends or grandchildren.

Our second action area covered the establishment of sustainable on-demand shuttle services [1]. These combine the benefits of public transport, such as environmental friendliness, pooling possibility and cost consciousness, with those of owning a vehicle like flexibility and comfort [20]. Pooling services offer mobility for older persons or persons in need of assistive devices as well as for other user groups as explored above. Compared to other sharing services like car sharing or bike sharing, on-demand shuttles offer more flexibility and provide a wider service range with better accessible vehicles [1, 21]. Yet, the associated time and cost aspects need to be considered. To attract new user groups to such (paratransit) shuttle services, individual rides should not take more time than a private car or any other transport opportunity available.

As stated before, the fares should be integrated in the prevailing public transport tariff systems [1] and furthermore should be lower than the taxi fares to provide pari passu access to all customer segments alike. The immense cost factor of shuttle services being available in all areas of a region [17] will most likely be reduced with the introduction of autonomous vehicles. Self-driving cars enhance individual mobility of persons who cannot drive or operate a car [22], as space currently occupied by steering wheel, pedals and gear stick can be made available for assistive technology [1]. Nevertheless, tariffs should be fair and affordable, in order to avoid a two-tier society, where marginalized persons are excluded from mobility services.

Thirdly, when discussing accessibility of transport services [1], we found that besides physical constraints, the digital accessibility of a transport system and its offerings is another important factor [23]. Schreder et al. [24] point out that even ticket vending machine functionalities and interfaces can drastically reduce accessibility to public transport. Additionally, a wide spectrum of apps, providing different pieces of information and service at varying digital accessibility levels, are important. However, some of these service offerings have not taken into consideration that people with impairments or minor digital experience might not be able to use these services due to their constraints [1].

When researching mobility assistance, a wide field for analysis opens up, including mobility issues from within one's own home to the independent travelling across neighborhoods and cities. Meurer et al. [15] have summarized various technological inventions and AAL solutions that are available for older adults as well as for people with sensory and/or physical impairments: Walking aids of any kind, skeletons, GPS equipped walkers, apps that guide through neighborhoods or emergency services for people who get lost. Obviously, cars and other means of transportation have become smarter too. These innovations are predominantly aiming at enhancing accessibility of places, increasing of people's mobility, navigation, safety, and security in mobility.

People remain reluctant however, when it comes to car and ride sharing, as this could have a negative impact on older adult's independence and autonomy [15].

Besides the issue of accessibility, Lavadinho [12] claims awareness for an often-ignored issue in the context of the public transportation debate. She discusses the interrelation between different public transportation services, as already discussed earlier, in optimally adapted networks. She also reflects upon the accessibility of transportation hubs. In this setting, providing "walk-friendly environments" is the responsibility of the transport authorities and should not be underestimated in its relevance for planners and decision makers: "Well, for one reason, public transport clients are walkers, first and foremost" [12]. Though her focus lays on the 'in-between-mile', her research reveals some important insights also for the 'first-' and 'last-mile' discussion. She puts the concept of the 'economy of speed' vis-a-vis the 'economy of place' [12]. The latter guarantees different user groups' satisfaction along the line of accessibility in terms of functionality, e.g. clear signage, services and infrastructure, like seating opportunities. The TransitCenter foundation too, stresses the importance of the mode of walking when accessing public transport stations [25]. We suggest these factors to be considered within intermodal transport systems, i.e. when changing from public transport lines to sharing or shuttle services in transport hubs.

When reflecting on these three quality-related action areas, our integrative view on transport systems, their customers and interlinking components among each other, expands into a transport ecosystem. Due to technological developments, individualized mobility patterns, new transport modes and options, and innovative business models new mobility services appear. As described by Litman [26], in order to fulfill todays mobility demand, transport systems are especially in need of new forms of cooperation between private and public transport operators (e.g. public transport providers and car sharing operators, PT-contractors and paratransit operators etc.), while the role of transport infrastructure management- and public authorities continuously changes and develops. Our shift in perception interweaves the "old school" transport system thinking with the chances and opportunities of new mobility services in a user-focused multi-stakeholder environment, taking into consideration ecological, social and economic frameworks and conditions.

4   Communication and Information Needs

More and more cities promote themselves as 'smart'; be it in the area of economy, governance, living or mobility. Smart mobility is about sustainability, inclusive services, and safe as well as secure mobility systems. Full use of ICT has become an indispensable must when providing mobility in a smart manner. In their study Bifulco et al. [27] confirm that "ICT is a tool for mobility because it can facilitate the use of public transport by providing logistical information, and it can even encourage a switch between different methods of transportation" [27]. Furthermore, they also stress the importance of apps facilitating smooth and uninterrupted journeys, real time information and flexibility. Apps also allow integrating information from different service providers.

As stated before [1], the digital transformation in the transport industry has become an important factor when it comes to the accessibility of mobility services [23]. Buying a ticket successfully increasingly is a question of having the right app stored and operational on your mobile devices. At the same time information becomes readily available, more and more complex, and options manifold. Above all, vending machines, which are currently accepted to be a requirement for public transport, can actually drastically reduce accessibility to public transport [24].

With ongoing digitization, both public transport operators as well as providers of shared services and their customers use the same mobile applications. Customers are informed in real-time, get navigation hints when arriving in a transportation hub, etc. These apps enable access to service offers beyond the pure mobility [23]. The wide spectrum of apps, which provide different pieces of information and services at varying digital accessibility levels, clearly improve the travel experience but also cause additional hassle and barriers. Not all customers are equally experienced and capable to use and interact with apps [1].

Nevertheless, access to communication and information channels is an important asset for all customers within a transport ecosystem. The "mobility2know" project [28] gives important insights into the quality of information customers would expect to know about a mobility service; even though from a technology usage point of view, this might no longer be relevant. Depending on the social situation and the physical environment, as well as the housing situation and location (combined depicted as so called mobility milieus), mobility behavior and therefore mobility information needs vary [28]. This also has to be taken into consideration, when designing accessible mobility solutions within a transport ecosystem. Besides, as pointed out in other ecosystem-related research in the AAL domain, trust as a key concern in the digital debate [29, 30] must not be neglected. Trust in the transportation service industry is not limited to fiath in punctuality and guaranteed connections. It is about relying on trustworthy options to access and book mobility services, on secured payment systems and on operators who enhance mobility, especially on the Last Mile. We strongly argue [1] that both centralizing and enriching the digital information available as well as integrating the ticketing and booking services of all mobility modes into a single accessible digital solution built on Universal Design principles [31] and the WCAG 2.0 Guidelines [32] would foster personal mobility for older adults and persons with disabilities. The customer group of the younger generation definitely would appreciate the digital transformation. Yet, only a smart integration of digital and non-digital information available would remove barriers to mobility.

While in Switzerland the population is well served by sharing services, customers are limited in their choice of destinations and are facing higher prices because of the lack of integration into a unified tariff model across city or canton boundaries. "People living in the outskirts of Zurich City might be better off searching for a transport service in the neighboring community or even the canton itself than with the cities' mobility services" [1]. By providing proper integrated and digital and non-digital information, access and payment within a unified tariff system, urban shuttle services are opened up to a wider audience, instead of creating parallel systems to public transport, as described by Neumann [7].

5   The Role of Shuttle Services and Paratransit

In order to enhance Last Mile mobility of older adults and persons with disabilities, we proposed the integration of (medical) shuttles into the public transport network [1]. Following the approach of previous sections, we expand our perspective on demand-driven paratransit towards other customers segments and their role within an urban transport ecosystem.

When investigating paratransit, there is a particularly interesting aspect: In European countries, like Austria and Switzerland, paratransit describes medical shuttles fulfilling the transport needs of persons with physical or psychological impairments. In contrast, African and Asian countries understand paratransit as a motorized transport service for all commuters within an urban area [7, 33], not focusing on needs of older adults or persons with disabilities. Yet, for the purpose of our work, paratransit is to describe those transport services, which are specifically organized and equipped to meet the needs of commuters with physical or mental disabilities.

The core business of paratransit operators, such as the Wiener Lokalbahnen Verkehrsdienste in Vienna, is the transportation of persons with reduced physical or mental abilities for work, school or medical purposes as well as leisure activities [21]. Paratransit services are, of course, also available in rural areas; there they are mostly offered to older adults [34]. Due to opening and business hours not only of workplaces, but also of schools and medical centers, paratransit shuttle services are concentrated in the mornings and in the evenings on workdays too. Above all, they do passenger pooling [17]. Like in public transport, the transport volume is lower during non-peak times of the day as well as during weekends and public holidays. One would think that paratransit shuttle services therefore should rather be offered in the non-productive times. We would however argue that similar passenger frequency in public transport and paratransit shuttles could be employed in a mutually beneficial way. In times when reduced service frequency and longer intervals are provided by public transport, an integrated paratransit operator would enable the replacement of the larger vehicles with more cost efficient shuttles. Moreover, it is in particular the Last Mile transport that can be covered by paratransit shuttles [1].

This, however, requires close collaboration and a comprehensive integration of the (medical) shuttle services into the public transport system [1]. By doing so, the current transport systems could be expanded to meet the needs of transport ecosystems. New stakeholders on both sides, provider and customer side, would be integrated. Such a transport ecosystem would also need to deal with new sources and qualities of information, with different service qualities and various means of transportation. Only through adequate digital platforms would the customer's experiences of planning, booking and paying become a fully accessible and manageable experience, without risks of loss of control. In addition, other operational aspects will need to be changed. The staff needs to be aware of their customers with special needs, of different payment modes, as well as (flexible and varying) pick-up and drop-off points for pooled rides. In this context, without doubt, digitization is and will be a pre-eminent driver and enabler.

Another important aspect is the need for some sort of service level agreement between public transport and paratransit operators. The proposed integration into the tariff system [1] needs to support the business goals of both parties. Otherwise, the risk of paratransit only covering the most profitable routes would arise [7], creating a "cannibalization effect" [35] between the operators. Therefore, it is important to stress, that the proposed integration of shuttles into the transport system [1] is an expansion of the paratransit operator's role beyond its core business. On one hand, covering the Last Mile transport only would force non-profitable operations onto paratransit businesses. On the other hand, it would exclude those passengers from transport, who are in need of additional service for the full transport required by their physical or mental state. Additionally, it has to be considered, that only if public transport accessibility is increased continuously, a sustainable and accessible transport system with on-demand shuttles can be established and maintained [17].

Schiefelbusch [36] investigated the involvement of volunteers in public transport in Germany, stressing the need for more flexibility and the reduction of costs. In addition, he concluded that rural and periurban areas are lacking a sufficient and dense transportation service network. In his understanding specific transport needs can be best serviced in an urbanized context. Here different and more transport providers operate. He clearly supports the respective claims by Glaeser [10]. Nevertheless, Stiefelbusch [36] criticizes that most transport logics hardly ever consider the customer needs with respect to their travel preferences. Moreover, independent from the spatial reference (urban, suburban or periurban), we can widely observe a need to foster the development of flexible and user-friendly services. This could be amended by volunteer service offers. Collaboration between public and private and/or volunteer providers however, is only successfully accepted and trusted, when it is well known, promoted and made accessible to the public [36].

6 Policy Needs and Recommendations

As concluded in our previous work, an open and interoperable digital system for the integration of technologically ready partners should be fostered by public authorities, while creating incentives to enable and offer accessible transport services [1]. Based on "their mission to provide mobility instead of maximizing profit, public transport operators can foster a unified and impartial integration of services into an interoperable and open digital platform, to be accessed by customers through a single user interface, i.e. a mobile App or a responsive website" [1]. We argue, this not only fosters the integration of different services and service providers but also makes public transportation more attractive and promotes it as a valid alternative to motorized individual transportation. In parallel, public transportation authorities should take the lead in setting the standards for accessible transportation. From a customer's point of view, the better integrated a transportation system is, the smoother the travel planning and the mobility itself become. We should critically assess the question whether public or volunteer based transportation services are more appropriate and efficient in serving the different customer needs.

In this context, Schiefelbusch [36] discusses the volunteer-based paratransit services in contrast to public transportation. He criticizes the lack of integration of user perspectives when developing public transport systems. He describes the volunteer-based paratransit system being a bottom-up service, tackling local mobility needs. These are the drivers for developing individualized and localized solutions. Similarly, Neven et al. [17] report that in the Flanders Region, Belgium, paratransit services originate from local ad hoc needs. In contrast, public transport is planned and operated based on mass transportation needs, driven by policies, urban development and occupancy rate.

Transportation policies and the development of a transportation ecosystem have to take into consideration that mobility is "actually not a matter of only providing transport. It is embedded in discourses of community life, social needs, preventing exclusion, maintaining and securing local identity" [36]. So, the digital integration of different service providers is only one aspect among others. In order to provide mobility in a transport ecosystem, additional measures must be taken in order to promote the services and to make them sustainable.

Participating in a transport ecosystem, which most likely would be dominated by public service providers, guarantees private and/or volunteer mobility service providers better marketing and operation with an umbrella branding. The individual brand identities must not be given up though. Such a common umbrella brand with established public and private transport offerings would have various positive effects for mobility services and their customers. It can be expected that in future travelling becomes even cheaper and smoother. As the specialized service for people with impairments will no longer only be provided by specialized and clearly branded service providers, but will be integrated in an overall service package, stigmatization of such users will also be reduced. Most notably trust in the service will increase. Trust in the brand of public transport operators in Switzerland and Austria is generally high and can thereby be leveraged towards the services of other providers. In summary, by visibly integrating paratransit into the transport ecosystem as a service to be used by everyone under a common umbrella brand, social inclusion of people with impairments and older adults is enhanced, beyond the cost-saving effects already described by Neven et al. [17].

Joining forces in mobility services and branding strategies, operators can pave their ways towards true Mobility-as-a-Service (MaaS) offerings. MaaS alliances and the respective projects and initiatives have arisen all over the world: Europe, USA, Canada, Australia and Asia [37]. MaaS, so the alliance, not only facilitates the access to mobility but it "should be the best value proposition, by helping them meet their mobility needs and solve the inconvenient parts of individual journeys as well as the entire system of mobility services" [37]. Furthermore, linking to what we discussed earlier, MaaS services are successfully developed and implemented along the line of new business models. Hoadley [38] claims that with MaaS personal mobility needs are best satisfied. Successful MaaS initiatives are, among others, digital pathfinders. Naturally, the importance of ICT to the transport industry is not new. When it comes to the individual mobility, from a technology point of view, various technological innovations, support people in using transportation systems [39]. Besides, smart navigation systems and online, real-time travel information, word processors to reduce the typing barrier etc. are in use as well as so-called smartcards, which guarantee free access to all means of transportation within the mobility service as well as a reduction of costs [39]. However, unifying access to various means of transportation is only the first step towards an overall MaaS service. Hoadley [38] summarizes four requirements for a successfully realized MaaS initiative. First, mass transportation services will not cease to exist, but they will need to adapt to changing requirements with respect to customer expectations and new technological possibilities. Second, service is best provided when you know your customer, when you know what each partner in the transport ecosystem is contributing. Data, which is available and accessible in real time, helps the customer to optimize services, routes, schedules. Digital platforms are considered a key to a successful implementation of superior business models and mobility services. Third, trust is a key concern in the new business relationships. This applies even more when customers no longer directly approach service providers and when the services are promoted and sold by other partners within the transport ecosystem. Fourth, marketing is key, as customers will no longer buy a train ticket to go from A to B but will optimize their overall service experience provided by different partners. Besides improved accessibility, the extension of mobility services into the suburban and peri-urban areas, the reduction of costs, and the integration of different customer group into the transportation ecosystem are advantages of smart MaaS projects.

There are various app and platform solutions for MaaS available. For instance, an app that reduces travel costs, as only the actual travel distances is paid for. "lezzgo" is promoted by the Swiss train company BLS. Customers no longer buy fixed-price tickets [40]. With the HaCon Kids App "VBB jump", in Berlin-Brandenburg, Germany, children are supported in their door to door travelling. Up to eight destinations can be planned in advance. When children miss a bus or take the wrong route, the app is informing their parents in real time. This app was co-developed with children [41]. In Oxford, a demand-responsive bus services was recently introduced. Via a "PickMeUp" app customers can request a pick-up at a virtual bus stop within a clearly defined service area [42]. In summary, in partnerships of different providers, customers would profit from a multimodal and intermodal transportation mode. However, Hoadley [38] clearly stresses: "Given the different circumstances in different cities and regions, it seems unlikely that a single MaaS model would be universally applicable."

In contrast to the new possibilities of the fast changing digital technologies - with the app and platform solutions - the actual transport technologies seem to change relatively slowly. This difference in pace will become critical when industry and suppliers move beyond telematics for car-2-car and car-2-X communication as well as autonomous driving [43] towards fully integrated transportation technologies [39]. When reaching this point, policies and road infrastructure will be required to be "smart" as well.

The developments in digitization ensure that both availability and accessibility to means of transportation are improved. Yet, progress in digitization implies the potential to outrace the actual implementation of transport ecosystems. Therefore, transport operators are required to enlarge the scope and their perspective of their core business providing mobility. While physical infrastructure and vehicle change happens slowly, operators need to accept methods and concepts like agile management, as well as technologies such as autonomous driving, in order to become more flexible and to adapt faster to shifting customer needs.

Nevertheless, even though very promising innovations in autonomous shuttles are already introduced in some cities and smaller communities, these will neither be sufficient nor will it be fast enough to solve all the challenges most European countries face. Connecting urban, suburban, periurban and rural communities sufficiently and tackle the problem of integrating people with very different mobility needs at present is best achieved with a holistic approach and by fostering public-private partnerships beyond the pure focus on transport automation [44].

7   Conclusion

In this article, we deepened and expanded our research on demand-driven mobility, covering five action areas proposed in our previous work [1]. We outlined that needs for and gains of enhanced (Last Mile) mobility of older adults and persons with disabilities align with those of marginalized persons, as well as children and adolescents. To ensure maximization of effects on personal mobility, we reviewed our analysis on Last Mile transport services and delved into information and communication needs of the customer segments. Based on our findings, we re-evaluated and deepened our previous position on the role of paratransit shuttles and policy making in this spectrum.

As public transport accessibility is increasing, on-demand paratransit shuttles are becoming an important, yet sustainable [17] component of the transport ecosystem. Fostering cooperation and umbrella branding activities, as well as opening up to new trends in technological developments, Last Mile transport service offers become more trustworthy and integrate into real MaaS solutions. By opening paratransit towards the general public within the transport ecosystem, stigmatization of customers with disabilities should be reduced, while social inclusion is enhanced.

Given these explored potentials, we propose the pilot operation of modern, accessible and ICT-supported on-demand transport service, covering Last Mile transport as well as end-to-end transport, integrated into a public transport ecosystem. Those pilots will demonstrate the mutual benefits of public transport service operators and on-demand transportation providers, which can be forwarded to their customers, supporting the achievement of a fair, available, accessible, affordable, and efficient transport ecosystem.

References

1. Ruscher, S., Kofler, A., Neumayer, V., Renat, J.: Intermodal transport systems as a chance to enhance first mile and last mile mobility of older adults and persons with disabilities - position paper on action areas for accessible urban and suburban transport. In: Bamidis, P., Ziefle, M., Maciaszek, L. (eds.) Proceedings of the 4th International Conference on Information and Communication Technologies for Ageing Well and e-Health (ICT4AWE 2018), pp. 200–208. SCITEPRESS – Science and Technology Publications, Lda, Portugal (2018)

2. European Commission: Proposal for a Directive of the European Parliament and of the Council on the approximation of the laws, regulations and administrative provisions of the Member States as regards the accessibility requirements for products and services (2015). http://eur-lex.europa.eu/legal-content/EN/TXT/?uri=COM:2015:0615:FIN. Accessed 27 July 2018

3. Shaheen, S., Guzman, S., Zhang, H.: Bikesharing in Europe, the Americas, and Asia: past, present, and future. Transp. Res. Rec.: J. Transp. Res. Board **2143**, 159–167 (2010)

4. Edyburn, D.: Would you recognize universal design for learning if you saw it? Ten propositions for new directions for the second decade of UDL. Learn. Disabil. Q. **33**(1), 33–41 (2010)

5. Ruscher, S., Burger, J., Sauli, E., Kofler, A.: Implementing WCAG and ISO 9241 in AAL software applications-a case study. In: 2nd IET International Conference on Technologies for Active and Assisted Living (TechAAL 2016), pp. 1–6. IET, London (2016)

6. Wobbrock, J., Kane, S., Gajos, K., Harada, S., Froehlich, J.: Ability-based design: Concept, principles and examples. ACM Trans. Accessible Comput. (TACCESS) **3**(3) (2011). Article 9

7. Neumann, A.: A paratransit-inspired evolutionary process for public transit network design. Epubli (2014)

8. Lubitow, A., Rainer, J., Bassett, S.: Exclusion and vulnerability on public transit: experiences of transit dependent riders in Portland. Oregon. Mobilities **12**(6), 924–937 (2017)

9. Ruscher, S., Jäger, B., Huber, F., Bertel, D.: Age-related safety and security – developing a novel threat and risk model for older adults. In: Piazolo, F., Schlögl, S. (eds.) Innovative Lösungen für eine alternde Gesellschaft. Konferenzbeiträge der SMARTER LIVES 16, 29 November 2016, Innsbruck, pp. 12–19. Pabst Science Publishers, Lengerich (2018)

10. Glaeser, E., Kahn, M., Rappaport, J.: Why do the poor live in cities? The role of public transportation. J. Urban Econ. **63**(1), 1–24 (2008)

11. Quodomine, R.: Further research into using geographic principles to analyze public transportation in the USA and maximize the concept of induced transit. In: Sustainable Urban Transport, pp. 121–147. Emerald Group Publishing Limited (2015)

12. Lavadinho, S.: Public transport infrastructure and walking: gearing towards the multimodal city. In: Walking: Connecting Sustainable Transport with Health, pp. 167–186. Emerald Publishing Limited (2017)

13. Schrenk, M., et al.: Bus Stop 3.0 - Bushaltestelle der Zukunft. Eine Forschungsstudie innerhalb des Impulsprogrammes ways2go – Technologien für sich wandelnde Mobilitäts-bedürfnisse/1. Ausschreibung. CEIT ALANOVA gemeinnützige GmbH, Schwechat, Austria (2010)

14. Stone, M., Faulkner, G., Mitra, R., Buliung, R.: The freedom to explore: examining the influence of independent mobility on weekday, weekend and after-school physical activity behaviour in children living in urban and inner-suburban neighbourhoods of varying socioeconomic status. Int. J. Behav. Nutr. Phys. Activity, **11**(1) (2014). Article 5

15. Meurer, J., Stein, M., Randall, D., Wulf, V.: Designing for way-finding as practices – a study of elderly people's mobility. Int. J. Hum Comput Stud. **115**, 40–51 (2018)

16. Stadt Wien: Bevölkerung nach Altersgruppen, Geschlecht und Gemeindebezirken 2016 (2016). https://www.wien.gv.at/statistik/bevoelkerung/tabellen/bevoelkerung-alter-geschl-bez.html. Accessed 27 July 2018

17. Neven, A., Braekers, K., Declercq, K., Wets, G., Janssens, D., Bellemans, T.: Assessing the impact of different policy decisions on the resource requirements of a demand responsive transport system for persons with disabilities. Transp. Policy **44**, 48–57 (2015)

18. VBZ Fahrplan. https://www.stadt-zuerich.ch/vbz/de/index/fahrplan.html. Accessed 27 July 2018

19. Marconi, D., Schad, H.: Mobilität in den ländlichen Räumen (Report). Bundesamt für Raumentwicklung, Bern (2016)
20. Huß, S., Frick, C., Keck, M.: Erneuerung der städtischen Mobilität. Wie kann ein Shuttle-System den kompletten motorisierten Individualverkehr in Hamburg ersetzen?. flinc GmbH, Darmstadt (2016)
21. Wiener Lokalbahnen Verkehrsdienste Homepage. http://www.verkehrsdienste.at/. Accessed 27 July 2018
22. Litman, T.: Autonomous Vehicle Implementation Predictions. Victoria Transport Policy Institute, USA (2017)
23. Giampapa, J., Steinfeld, A., Teves, E., Dias, M., Rubinstein, Z.: Accessible Transportation Technologies Research Initiative (ATTRI): State of the Practice Scan. Robotics Institute, Carnegie Mellon University, USA (2017)
24. Schreder, G., Siebenhandl, K., Mayr, E., Smuc, M.: The Ticket Machine Challenge: Social Inclusion by Barrier-free Ticket Vending Machines. Generational Use of New Media, pp. 129–148 (2016)
25. TransitCenter: Who's On Board 2016. What Today's Riders Teach Us About Transit That Works. TransitCenter, New York, USA (2016)
26. Litman, T.: Introduction to Multi-Modal Transportation Planning. Victoria Transport Policy Institute, USA (2014)
27. Bifulco, F., Tregua, M., Amitrano, C., D'Auria, A.: ICT and sustainability in smart cities management. Int. J. Public Sector Manage. 29(2), 132–147 (2016)
28. Dangschat, J., Mayr, R.: Der Milieu-Ansatz in der Mobilitätsforschung. Technische Universität Wien, Vienna, Austria (2012)
29. Teles, S., Bertel, D., Kofler, A., Ruscher, S. Paúl, C.: A multi-perspective view on AAL stakeholders' needs - a user-centred requirement analysis for the active advice European project. In: Röcker, C., O'Donoghue, J., Ziefle, M., Maciaszek, L., Molloy, W. (eds.) Proceedings of the 3rd International Conference on Information and Communication Technologies for Ageing Well and e-Health (ICT4AWE 2017), pp. 104–116. SCITEPRESS – Science and Technology Publications, Lda, Portugal (2017)
30. Teles, S., Kofler, Andrea Ch., Schmitter, P., Ruscher, S., Paúl, C., Bertel, D.: ActiveAdvice: a multi-stakeholder perspective to understand functional requirements of an online advice platform for AAL products and services. In: Röcker, C., O'Donoghue, J., Ziefle, M., Maciaszek, L., Molloy, W. (eds.) ICT4AWE 2017. CCIS, vol. 869, pp. 168–190. Springer, Cham (2018). https://doi.org/10.1007/978-3-319-93644-4_9
31. National Disability Authority: The 7 Principles (2014). http://universaldesign.ie/What-is-Universal-Design/The-7-Principles/. Accessed 27 July 2018
32. Cladwell, B., et al.: Web Content Accessibility Guidelines (WCAG) 2.0 (2008). https://www.w3.org/TR/WCAG20/. Accessed 27 July 2018
33. Tangphaisankun, A., Nakamura, F., Okamura, T.: Influences of paratransit as a feeder of mass transit system in developing countries based on commuter satisfaction. In: Proceedings of the Eastern Asia Society for Transportation Studies Vol. 7 (The 8th International Conference of Eastern Asia Society for Transportation Studies, 2009), p. 236. Eastern Asia Society for Transportation Studies (2009)
34. Bond, M., Brown, J., Wood, J.: Adapting to challenge: examining older adult transportation in rural communities. Case Stud. Transp. Policy 5(4), 707–715 (2017)
35. Bróg, W.: Switching to public transport. In: UITP Asia Pacific Congress, Melbourne (2000)
36. Schiefelbusch, M.: German experiences with volunteer-based paratransit and public transport. In: Paratransit: Shaping the Flexible Transport Future, pp. 77–102. Emerald Group Publishing Limited (2016)

37. MaaS Alliance Partner News. https://maas-alliance.eu/maas-news/partner-news/. Accessed 30 July 2018
38. Hoadley, S.: Mobility as a service: Implications for urban and regional transport. Discussion paper offering the perspective of Polis member cities and regions on Mobility as a Service (MaaS). In: Polis, vol. 9 (2017)
39. Metz, D.: Future transport technologies for an ageing society: practice and policy. In: Transport, Travel and Later Life, pp. 207–220. Emerald Publishing Limited (2017)
40. Lezzgo Hompage. https://www.lezzgo.ch/index-en.html. Accessed 30 July 2018
41. VBB jump - die App für Kinder. http://www.vbb.de/de/article/startseite/vbb-jump/jump/1782955.html. Accessed 30 July 2018
42. Intelligent Transport: Demand-responsive bus services have arrived in Oxford. https://www.intelligenttransport.com/transport-news/67878/demand-responsive-bus-services-oxford/. Accessed 30 July 2018
43. Ruscher, S., Jäger, B., Hillebrand, J., Karner, M.: A case study on imobility and police - involving public authorities in applied security research and creating a holistic technology classification system. In: 14th ESCAR Europe (2016)
44. Mendes, D.: Bind the gap: Resolving transit's first-and-last-mile challenge (2017). http://www.metro-magazine.com/technology/news/725677/bind-the-gap-resolving-transit-s-first-and-last-mile-challenge. Accessed 27 July 2018

Author Index

Printed in the United States
By Bookmasters